Neuroscience, Psychotherapy, and Clinical Pragmatism

This volume explores how the principles and values of pragmatic philosophy serve as orienting perspectives for critical thinking in contemporary psychotherapy and clinical practice.

Drawing on the contributions of William James and John Dewey, *Neuroscience, Psychotherapy, and Clinical Pragmatism* introduces a model of clinical pragmatism emphasizing the individuality of the person, open-ended dialogue, experiential learning, and the practical outcomes of ideas and methods. In a second part, chapters show how recent developments in neuroscience and interpersonal neurobiology deepen our understanding of change and growth in accord with the principles of clinical pragmatism. Finally, the volume reviews paradigms of psychotherapy across the psychodynamic, behavioral, cognitive, and humanistic traditions. Case studies show how the pluralist orientation of clinical pragmatism enlarges concepts of therapeutic action.

This text has been written for psychotherapists as well as scholars, educators, and trainees in the fields of psychiatry, clinical psychology, counseling, and social work.

William Borden teaches at the University of Chicago, USA, where he directs the post-graduate Fellowship Program in Psychodynamic Psychotherapy. He works in independent practice as a psychotherapist.

Psychoanalytic Explorations

Books in this series:

Neuroscience, Psychotherapy, and Clinical Pragmatism

Reflective Practice and Therapeutic Action

William Borden

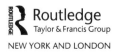

Routledge
Taylor & Francis Group

NEW YORK AND LONDON

First published 2021
by Routledge
52 Vanderbilt Avenue, New York, NY 10017

and by Routledge
2 Park Square, Milton Park, Abingdon, Oxon OX14 4RN

Routledge is an imprint of the Taylor & Francis Group, an informa business

Library of Congress Cataloging-in-Publication Data
Names: Borden, William, author.
Title: Neuroscience, psychotherapy, and clinical pragmatism : reflective
practice and therapeutic action / William Borden.
Description: New York : Routledge, 2021. |
Series: Psychoanalytic explorations |
Includes bibliographical references and index.
Identifiers: LCCN 2020040978 | ISBN 9781138825727 (hardback) |
ISBN 9781315739762 (ebook)
Subjects: LCSH: Neurosciences. | Psychotherapy.
Classification: LCC RC321 .B67 2021 | DDC 616.89/14--dc23
LC record available at https://lccn.loc.gov/2020040978

ISBN: 978-1-138-82572-7 (hbk)
ISBN: 978-0-367-70141-3 (pbk)
ISBN: 978-1-315-73976-2 (ebk)

Typeset in Galliard
by Taylor & Francis Books

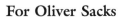

For Oliver Sacks

Contents

About the Author

William Borden, PhD, has taught courses on psychoanalysis, comparative psychotherapy, and human development at the University of Chicago for three decades, where he served as Associate Professor and Senior Lecturer in the School of Social Administration and Lecturer in the Department of Psychiatry. He directs the post-graduate Fellowship Program in Psychodynamic Psychotherapy at the University and works in independent practice as a clinician and consultant in Chicago. He is the author of *Contemporary Psychodynamic Theory and Practice* and other writings on a range of concerns, including the work of Donald Winnicott and the Independent Tradition in British psychoanalysis, narrative psychology, and stress and coping.

A Note to the Reader

> Each of us is a singular narrative, which is constructed, continually, unconsciously, by, through, and in us—through our perceptions, our feelings, our thoughts, our actions; and, not least, our discourse, our spoken narrations. Biologically, physiologically, we are not so different from each other; historically, as narratives—we are each of us unique.
>
> –Oliver Sacks

I had hoped that Oliver Sacks would be able to write the foreword for this account of psychotherapy and clinical pragmatism, but he died shortly after I began the project, seven months after he was diagnosed with metastatic liver cancer. Even so, he remains a presence in these pages. Over the years I have returned to his essays in my teaching, and his collections of case histories— "studies, stories" he called them—continue to deepen my appreciation of essential concerns in the practice of psychotherapy, documenting our capacities for change and growth following adversity and misfortune. His essay, "Neurology and the soul," published in 1990, helped me negotiate the gap between the "gray" of theory and the green and golden colors of life, as Goethe had put it, challenging students and clinicians to rediscover the richness of the phenomenal world of experience that defies classification or categorization—the world of the experiencing, active, living "I" that he captured so fully in the moving accounts of his practice. In a return to the tradition of the case history that had shaped understanding in the 19th century, Sacks emphasized the concrete particularity of people and lives and the crucial place of observation, empathy, and imagination in help and care.

When we met in 2002 we found that we shared a range of concerns, interests, and enthusiasms. Each of us had come to think of William James as an "essential other"—he spoke of him as "that adorable genius"—and we recounted the ways in which we called upon his concreteness of mind and pragmatic sensibilities as we carried out our clinical practice, he as a neurologist, I as a psychotherapist, ever suspicious of grand theory, searching for the "cash value" of ideas in the given case. "Like you," he wrote in a letter, "I find James a compass… I think I am on my fourth, fifth, n-th reading of the *Principles*," and he planned to reread *The Varieties of Religious Experience* shortly. Sacks reminded me that James brings the realms of neurophysiology and the transcendent together—"where they belong."

We continued to meet and correspond over the years, sharing accounts of our cases, clinical experience, reading (and re-reading), and we found ourselves returning to the writings of James, exploring points of connection between pragmatic philosophy, the science of mind, and the day to day practice of psychotherapy. He exemplified the values and principles that shape the account of clinical pragmatism I offer in this book, approaching the patient as a human subject first and last, engaging the "experiencing, active, living 'I'" (Sacks, 1984, p. 177).

In following a clinical pragmatism, as we will see, we do our best to understand the phenomenal world of subjective experience, taking account of the richness and the complexity and the contingency of the human situation, coming to appreciate what it means to be a unique individual. "We have, each of us, a life story... Biologically, physiologically, we are not so different from each other; historically, as narratives—we are each of us unique" (Sacks, 1985, p. 110). It is crucial to listen to our patients and to imagine their worlds, bridging observation, conversation, empathy, and careful description with the collective wisdom of our professions and the findings of scientific research as we work to understand what is the matter and what carries the potential to help.

The reader will note that I use the first person pronoun "we" throughout the book. Paradoxically, our focus on the concrete particularity of the individual deepens our appreciation of the ways in which we are all "much more simply human than otherwise," as Harry Stack Sullivan proposed in his "one genus postulate," whether we happen to find ourselves in the role of the patient or the clinician (Sullivan, 1953, p. 32). Although many psychotherapists use the term "client," I prefer the term "patient." The Latin root, from "patientem," meaning "suffering," "bearing," and "enduring," most fully captures my sense of the vulnerability, resilience, and steadfastness I rediscover in the day to day practice of psychotherapy.

William Borden
University of Chicago
Chicago, IL
July 14, 2020

References

Sacks, O. (1984). *A leg to stand on*. New York: Simon and Schuster.
Sacks, O. (1985). *The man who mistook his wife for a hat*. New York: Simon & Schuster.
Sacks, O. (1990). Neurology and the soul. *New York Review of Books*, Nov. 22.
Sullivan, H. S. (1953). *The interpersonal theory of psychiatry*. New York: Norton.

Acknowledgements

I write not as a scholar or researcher but as a psychotherapist and teacher, and I am deeply grateful to the patients, students, and colleagues who have shared their experience over the decades, enriching my life beyond measure, enlarging my appreciation of essential concerns in help and care. We hand one another along, as we carry out our work, and it remains a special pleasure to continue the conversation.

I have expressed my debt of gratitude to Oliver Sacks in the dedication and the Note to the Reader. Another physician, Robert Coles, remains a steadfast presence in my teaching and practice, urging us to call upon our novelists, poets, and artists as we negotiate the abstractions of theory and the generalizations of empirical research, rediscovering the concrete particularity of the individual and the workings of fate, circumstance, and fortune that shape the course of our lives. Our conversations have deepened my appreciation of the crucial role of the humanities in clinical training as we consider our experience of challenge, suffering, limitation, and loss, searching for meaning and purpose.

I first found myself speaking of a "clinical pragmatism" three decades ago as I introduced the work of Donald Winnicott in my seminar on the Independent Tradition in British psychoanalysis, moved by unexpected points of connection with the work of William James and John Dewey. As we return to their writings we rediscover a generosity of spirit that sponsors the presence of thinkers across divergent schools of thought, joining the realms of science and the humanities, challenging us to explore shared concerns and expand ways of attending, understanding, and acting.

My teaching continued to provide occasions to engage the concerns I explore in this book. As we entered the "Decade of the Brain," a growing number of students and colleagues wanted to consider the implications of recent developments in the science of mind for therapeutic practice, and I introduced a seminar on neuroscience and psychotherapy. Following advances in clinical neuroscience and pharmacology, some of my colleagues in the fields of psychiatry and neurology had predicted that biomedical models of explanation and treatment would supersede the practice of psychotherapy. Ironically, we would find that converging lines of study in the fields of neuroscience only reaffirm the crucial role of the therapeutic practices we have carried out for more than a century.

A range of thinkers and researchers across the fields of neuroscience have shaped my understanding of brain and mind. I draw on the contributions of Iain McGilchrist, Allan Schore, Daniel Siegel, and Louis Cozolino in my treatment of interpersonal neurobiology, and I am ever grateful for the clarity of mind they bring to their conceptual syntheses and reviews of empirical findings. David Brendel, trained as a psychiatrist and philosopher, has helped me join scientific understanding and humanistic values through his accounts of clinical pragmatism.

Over the years many colleagues and friends have expanded my understanding of the ideas and concerns I explore here, including Sharon Berlin on the science of mind and psychotherapy; Christopher Bollas on Winnicott and the Independent Tradition in British psychoanalysis; the late Bertram Cohler on narrative psychology; Andrew Davis on the physician-patient relationship; the late Jarl Dyrud on psychoanalysis and behavior therapy; Irene Elkin on the history of psychotherapy research; Mark Epstein on the trauma of everyday life and mindfulness; the late Miriam Elson and Jill Gardner on self psychology; Ingrid Gould on the healing functions of nature; the late Stephen Mitchell on relational psychoanalysis; Paul Wachtel on therapeutic communication, and Froma Walsh on resilience. Kate Edgar, who collaborated with Oliver Sacks as editor and researcher for more than 30 years, remains a supporting presence as I return to his essays and letters. Allen Heinemann, my spouse, working as a researcher, teacher, and clinician in the field of rehabilitation medicine, has deepened my understanding of trauma, healing, and recovery.

Thanks and more thanks to Peter Mudd, my therapist of three decades, who brought his own energy of mind and pragmatism to his close reading and editing of the manuscript. James Clark, Dennis McCaughan, Linda Tartof, and Karen Teigiser, old souls and collaborators on many projects, read sections, discussed concerns, and made critical suggestions.

I am ever grateful for the support and encouragement of many colleagues and friends over the years, including Marian Alexander, Jay Ammerman, Paula Ammerman, David Barford, Deborah Barford, Kevin Barrett, Theresa Brancaccio, James Brandt, the late Nancy Brandt, Michael Brannon, Ruth Brannon, Anne Brody, Margaret Brown, Mary Bunn, Don Camp, Jeff Carlson, Doug Culbert, Kelli Fitzgerald, Matt Fitzgerald, Wayne Gordon, Hannah Gordon, Kurt Hansen, Billy Hayes, Nina Helstein, the late Peter Homans, Robert Hsiung, Fruman Jacobson, Marian Jacobson, Maureen Kelly, Denis Keppeler, Tom LaClair, Jeanne LaDuke, Flora Lazar, Linda Levin, Alan Levy, the late Jason McVicker, Joel Morris, Scott Petersen, Elizabeth Peterson, Steve Peterson, Philip River, Sandra Rubovits, Robert Spitz, Jason Stell, Carol Stukey, Betty Sweetland, Bill Sweetland, David Tartof, and Hazel Vespa. I thank my colleagues at the University of Chicago for their support over the years, especially Summerson Carr, Rob Chaskin, Jessica Darrow, Colleen Grogan, Sydney Hans, Julia Henley, Edward Lawlor, Jeanne Marsh, Stanley McCracken, Harold Pollack, William Pollak, Gina Samuels, John Schuerman, Deborah Gorman-Smith, and Miwa Yasui. I thank Maureen Stimming for her ongoing support of our post-graduate fellowship program in psychodynamic psychotherapy, now in its 20th year, and my co-instructors, Carol Ganzer and Denise Davis.

My deepest thanks to Allen, my partner of 35 years. We continue to rediscover the wonder and sweetness of this life, and I am ever grateful for his love, steadfastness, support, and challenge. He joins me in loving thanks to our families.

I thank my editor at Routledge, Elsbeth Wright, and her editorial assistant, AnnaMary Goodall, for their thought, care, and support over the course of the project.

Except in the case of well-known figures introduced by first and last names, I have changed names and altered identifying details in order to protect privacy.

I am grateful for permission to expand earlier accounts of pragmatic philosophy and the relational paradigm in psychoanalytic thought.

Brief sections of Chapter 1 and an earlier version of a case study in Chapter 9 have been adapted from W. Borden (2013) Experiments in adapting to need: Pragmatism as orienting perspective in clinical social work, *Journal of Social Work Practice, 27*, 259–271. Adapted by permission of Routledge/Taylor and Francis Group.

Portions of Chapter 5 have been adapted from W. Borden (2009) *Contemporary psychodynamic theory and practice*, Chapters 12 and 13, New York: Oxford University Press; and W. Borden and J. Clark (2012) Contemporary psychodynamic theory, research, and practice: Implications for evidence-based intervention, in T. Rzepnicki, S. McCracken & H. Briggs (Eds.), *From task-centered social work to evidence-based and integrative practice* (pp. 65–88), New York: Oxford University Press. Adapted by permission of Oxford University Press

Introduction

You must bring out of each word its practical cash value, set it at work within the stream of your experience...

–William James

This book originates in my experience as a psychotherapist and teacher. I have worked as a clinician for four decades, and my teaching has provided ongoing occasions to explore the uses of theory in therapeutic practice—how divergent traditions and thinkers shape our understanding of what is the matter and what carries the potential to help, how we call upon different ideas and approaches as we negotiate the irreducible ambiguities and complexities of the clinical situation. Over the years I have come to appreciate the variety of ways in which we carry out what Donald Winnicott called "experiments in adapting to need," gathering "this and that, here and there," as he told his colleagues, creating original approaches from a range of perspectives in light of the concrete particulars of the given case (1945/1975, p. 145).[1]

In the course of our development as clinicians, I emphasize in my teaching, we must negotiate fundamental tensions between more pure conceptions of the therapeutic endeavor—more idealized versions of what we think of as help and care—and more pragmatic, provisional renderings of what we do as we carry out our work. Some of us search for an encompassing point of view that would promise to unify our understandings of people, problems in living, and therapeutic action. Certain thinkers offer moving accounts of the human situation and their sense of life, fashioning grand theories that followers regard as the foundations of therapeutic practice. In the rich tableau of the psychoanalytic tradition, for example, we find the drive psychologies of Sigmund Freud and Melanie Klein, the existential vision of Wilfred Bion, the self psychology of Heinz Kohut.

Other thinkers argue that the complexities and contingencies of the therapeutic encounter inevitably violate the integrity of our purist paradigms. Instead, they embrace a theoretical pluralism and exemplify the pragmatic attitude as they engage ideas and methods from a range of perspectives, steadfast in their focus on the particular circumstances of the clinical situation. C. G. Jung, Harry Stack Sullivan, and Winnicott bring a muscular pragmatism to their use of theory and technique. They speak to us in a distinctive voice and care deeply about ideas, but common sense and practical flexibility matter more than theoretical coherence as they negotiate the challenges of the clinical situation. Most important, they show in their case studies, is what works.

While many clinicians are trained in a single approach—nowadays usually a version of cognitive-behavioral therapy—most practitioners come to realize the limits of any particular model or thinker, finding that our grand theories inevitably fail us as we engage the realities of everyday practice. Although pure models of treatment are taught and tested in randomized controlled trials in academic training programs around the world, surveys continue to show that most psychotherapists endorse "eclecticism" as their fundamental orientation to practice. Unlike researchers, it would seem, practitioners seldom think of themselves as purists.

In our reviews of the clinical literature, however, we rarely find any discussion of the concerns, values, or principles that shape the ways in which therapists make use of different ideas and methods over the course of help and care. These are crucial matters as we consider the strengths and limits of divergent approaches and establish ways of working that are authentic and therapeutic, reflecting our voice and sensibility. In day to day practice, as Leston Havens cautioned in his classic account of comparative psychotherapy more than 40 years ago, what clinicians represent as "eclecticism" often lacks a conceptual rigor, perpetuating facile and unfocused ways of working, tending to "underplay differences" and "homogenize complexities" across the foundational schools of thought so that the powerful ideas and methods of different schools "lose their edge" (Havens, 1973/1987, p. 330).[2]

If we are to avoid the dogmatic embrace of a single paradigm or a willy-nilly eclecticism, I argue in this book, it is crucial to establish a point of view and to formulate basic principles and values that guide the ways we engage different theories, empirical findings, and technical procedures in a critically reflective practice. We need to be able to justify and defend what we say and do in light of the particular circumstances of the given case, the authority of our clinical experience, and the beliefs, values, and sensibilities that shape our ways of working. Otherwise we run the risk of purism or eclecticism by default, failing to realize the power and efficacy of different approaches in particular cases.

In Part I of this book I show how conceptions of pragmatism set forth in American philosophy serve as orienting perspectives for critical thinking in therapeutic practice, focusing our attention on essential concerns in the clinical situation. Drawing on the seminal contributions of William James and John Dewey, I review fundamental features of pragmatic thought, arguing that it offers important if largely unarticulated principles and ethical perspectives for therapeutic practice. I outline a working formulation of clinical pragmatism, emphasizing the importance of theoretical pluralism and comparative approaches to understanding; the practical outcomes of ideas in a given situation; and the crucial role of subjectivity, relationship, narrative, and experiential learning over the course of help and care. In following the values and principles of clinical pragmatism, as we will see, we work to understand the phenomenal realm of subjective experience and the distinctive character of people and lives, taking account of the richness, complexity, and contingency of the human situation, coming to appreciate what it means to be a unique individual.

***

The first generation of pragmatic philosophers drew on biology and psychology in developing their conceptions of mind, knowledge, and action in everyday life, and James and Dewey prefigure orienting ideas and concerns that have shaped the science of mind in our time. The pluralism of the pragmatic perspective, encompassing scientific and humanistic perspectives, allows us to think of ourselves as physical beings without recourse to a reductive materialism, joining the biological, psychological, and social realms of experience. I explore recent developments in the fields of neuroscience in Part II of the book and show how the orienting perspectives and empirical findings of interpersonal neurobiology deepen our appreciation of subjectivity, relationship, narrative, and therapeutic action in accord with the principles and values of clinical pragmatism.

Following the expansion of clinical neuroscience and pharmacology at the end of the 20th century, some scholars predicted that biomedical models of explanation and treatment would supersede the practice of psychotherapy. Ironically, recent lines of study in the science of mind only reaffirm the fundamental importance of established therapeutic practices in our efforts to bring about change and growth, emphasizing the crucial functions of the relationship and the varieties of experiential learning over the course of help and care. The research that emerged over the "decade of the brain" at the end of the 20th century has deepened our appreciation of the power of therapeutic practices we have carried out for more than a century.

Researchers have moved beyond the fundamental debate of nature versus nurture in their conceptions of development, and we continue to realize the ways in which brain and mind are shaped by a complex interplay of genetic action and experiential opportunities in the social surround. The brain is far more plastic than modern neuroscientists once believed, neither "hard-wired" nor fixed, and we increasingly appreciate the crucial role of relational life, narrative, various kinds of activity, and experiential learning in change and growth. Conceptual syntheses and research in the fields of neuroscience have strengthened the empirical foundations of psychotherapy, linking basic science to concepts of therapeutic action across the foundational schools of thought. Findings indicate that diverse forms of activity and learning carry the potential to change the brain throughout the life course, creating new neurons from neural stem cells and strengthening synaptic connections across existing networks, expanding the core structures and functions of the nervous system (Costandi, 2016; Doidge, 2015; Kandel, 1998, 2006, 2012, 2018; Sapolsky, 2017; Siegel, 2020).

The science of mind continues to enlarge our understanding of vulnerability and resilience across the course of life. From the perspective of neuroscience, we assume that genetic action, lapses in caretaking, restrictions of opportunity, and various kinds of traumatic experience potentially undermine the development of the brain and the emergence of self, compromising the growth and integration of neural networks, predisposing us to a range of vulnerabilities and problems in functioning that we encompass in our conceptions of psychopathology. Under-developed, under-integrated, or under-regulated networks are thought to perpetuate rigid or chaotic patterns of behavior (Cozolino, 2017; Kandel, 2018; Sapolsky, 2017; Schore, 2019a, 2019b; Siegel, 2020).

If we consider the neural substrates of the "talking cure," a fundamental task of psychotherapy is to generate experiential opportunities that reinstate developmental processes, restoring and strengthening the integration and regulation of neural functions believed to underlie our sense of self, well-being, and adaptive functioning. In this sense we understand psychotherapy as an enriching experience that enhances neuroplasticity and neural integration, altering the structure and function of the brain (Cozolino, 2017; Kandel, 1998, 2006, 2018; Schore, 2019a, 2019b; Solms, 2018a, 2018b). Reviews of research in the fields of neurogenetics, molecular biology, and brain imaging provide empirical support for these formulations, documenting changes in gene expression, neurotransmitter metabolism, and enduring modifications in synaptic plasticity following psychotherapy (Collerton, 2013; Cozolino, 2017; Glass, 2008; Kandel, 2018; Sapolsky, 2017; Schore, 2019b; Solms, 2018a, 2018b). The experiential changes that we see over the course of psychotherapy would appear to be closely linked to changes in the structure and function of the brain.

While we are at a very early stage in our understanding of the fundamental mechanisms that govern change and growth in psychotherapy—how and why it works—emerging accounts of development in neuroscience point to the crucial importance of pragmatic, flexible approaches that integrate shared elements as well as different forms of therapeutic action set forth in the psychodynamic, behavioral, cognitive, and humanistic paradigms of practice. Drawing on the developmental perspectives of interpersonal neurobiology, psychotherapy research findings, and clinical observation, we can identify core processes and domains of experience that would appear to be fundamental in fostering change, validating concepts of therapeutic action across the schools of thought.

Clinical scholars describe basic factors believed to operate in all forms of therapy, emphasizing the critical role of the therapeutic relationship and interactive experience, as well as specific methods developed within particular schools of thought, proposing that different approaches potentially engage different neuro-anatomical structures instrumental in our experience of bodily sensation, emotion, imagery, cognition, memory, and behavior. Research on the neurobiological correlates of psychotherapy is ongoing, but the orienting perspectives of neuroscience emphasize the need to consider multiple theories, therapeutic languages, and technical procedures as we carry out "experiments in adapting to need" and generate diverse forms of experiential learning thought to facilitate change and growth.

***

Although converging lines of study in the science of mind affirm the fundamental importance of theoretical pluralism and comparative approaches in therapeutic practice, many clinical training programs in psychiatry, psychology, counseling, social work and the other helping professions marginalize theory and embrace reductive models of evidence-based treatment, emphasizing mastery of skills and technical procedures rather than comparative study of clinical theories that provide conceptual foundations for critical thinking and "experiments in adapting to need." Without a solid grounding in the foundational theories of psychotherapy, I argue in this book, we run the risk of carrying out reductive, mechanized approaches to treatment by protocol, lacking conceptual foundations to negotiate the complexities and ambiguities of the clinical situation, failing to understand the elements we are trying to integrate and why. We may underestimate the potential benefits of different ways of working over the course of the therapeutic process, just as we may fail to appreciate the efficacy of more focused, circumscribed approaches to our practice. At root, as William James reminds us, theories are instruments, providing us with tools for critical thinking, methods for carrying out our practice, and justifications for our actions.

In light of these circumstances, the current moment seems right to reconsider what the foundational schools of psychotherapy offer us as we take account of recent developments in neuroscience and rethink concepts of therapeutic action. In Part III of the book I focus on paradigms of psychotherapy set forth in the psychodynamic, behavioral, cognitive, and humanistic traditions. I review concepts of therapeutic action that have shaped understanding and practice over the years, realizing that many clinicians have not had opportunities to explore the wider range of theories in the course of their training, and consider recent developments in the science of mind that deepen our understanding of change and growth in accord with the principles and values of clinical pragmatism. I hope that students and teachers of psychotherapy, researchers, and practitioners of different orientations will challenge the climate of parochialism and factionalism that has divided clinicians across the foundational schools of thought over the decades and deepen their appreciation of other perspectives, exploring shared concerns and different points of emphasis.

The critical root of theory, *theamai*, means "to behold," and the foundational schools of thought challenge us to deepen our powers of observation and imagination, enlarging ways of attending, understanding, speaking, and acting, bringing different points of emphasis to our practice. The ways in which we focus our attention shape the course and outcomes of the therapeutic process. As Ian McGilchrist emphasizes, attention is more than a cognitive function: "Attention changes *what kind of* a thing comes into being for us: in that way it changes the world" (2009, p. 28). The act of observation itself can be transformative, altering what is being observed. "Through the direction and nature of our attention," McGilchrist explains, "we prove ourselves to be partners in creation" (2009, p. 28). If each paradigm inevitably fails to capture the variety and complexity of human experience, all are crucial because they set forth distinct values, visions of reality, and therapeutic action, helping us appreciate the implications of different ideas by pressing them to their limits, reflecting the multiplicity of life itself (Borden, 2010, 2018; Messer, 2001; Messer & Kaslow, 2020; Safran & Messer, 1998; Strenger, 1997). Our therapeutic practice deserves all the rich variety of insight that we can bring to our understanding of what carries the potential to help.

As we will see, the pluralist orientation of clinical pragmatism preserves the distinct identities of the foundational schools of thought and makes the multiplicity of differing approaches a defining feature of therapeutic practice. In the closing chapter of the book I present two cases and consider the challenges we face as we engage the principles and values of clinical pragmatism. If pragmatic perspectives broaden the scope of understanding and strengthen critical thinking over the course of the therapeutic process, they place considerable demands on the practitioner. We must consider multiple theories, therapeutic languages, models, and methods, negotiating tensions between a particular approach and alternative points of view as we work to determine what is helpful in the concrete particularity of the clinical situation. As James describes the task: "You must bring out of each word its practical cash value, set it at work within the stream of your experience..." (James, 1907/1946, p. 53). The challenge is to establish an *open* practice that potentially encompasses a range of perspectives and yet preserves the distinctive presence and voice the clinician and the patient. I emphasize the importance of ongoing dialogue across the fields of neuroscience, the foundational schools of thought, and the humanities as we rediscover shared concerns and fundamental purposes in the varieties of therapeutic experience.

Notes

1 Donald Winnicott challenged orthodox conceptions of psychoanalysis, rejecting models of "standard psychotherapy," explaining that he carried out "experiments in adapting to need" in light of the particular circumstances, possibilities, and constraints of the given case; he describes his method and ways of working to his colleagues in the British Psycho-Analytic Society at the start of his first major talk, "Primitive emotional development" (1945/1975, p. 145).
2 The disadvantage of eclecticism is its lack of conceptual rigor. The Greek root of the term eclectic, *eklektikos*, means "selective." As Havens cautions, however, clinicians may find themselves engaging a limited range of ideas on the basis of their appeal rather than undertaking "the much more taxing matter of mastering all the methods of schools and discerning when to use them" in critical, focused ways of working (1973/1987, p. 330). He proposes pluralism as an alternative to eclecticism.

References

Borden, W. (2010). Taking multiplicity seriously, in W. Borden (Ed.), *Reshaping theory in contemporary social work practice: Toward a critical pluralism in clinical practice* (pp.3–27). New York: Columbia University Press.

Borden, W. (2018). Winnicott and the Independent Tradition in British psychoanalysis: Presence, voice, and therapeutic action. Invited Lecture, Fellows Program in Advanced Psychodynamic Psychotherapy, Dec. 14, University of Chicago, Chicago, IL.

Collerton, D. (2013). Psychotherapy and brain plasticity. *Frontiers in Psychology*, 4, 548.

Costandi, M. (2016). *Neuroplasticity*. Cambridge, MA: MIT Press.

Cozolino, L. (2017). *The Neuroscience of psychotherapy*, 3rd edn. New York: Norton.

Doidge, N. (2015). *The brain's way of healing*. New York: Viking.

Glass, R. M. (2008). Psychodynamic psychotherapy and research evidence: Bambi survives Godzilla. *Journal of the American Medical Association*, 300, 1587–1589.

Havens, L. (1973/1987). *Approaches to the mind: Movement of the psychiatric schools from sect to science*. Cambridge, MA: Harvard University Press.

James, W. (1907/1946). *Pragmatism*. New York: Longmans, Green.

Kandel, E. (1998). A new intellectual framework for psychiatry. *American Journal of Psychiatry*, 155 (4), 457–469.

Kandel, E. (2006). *In search of memory: The emergence of a new science of mind*. New York: Norton.

Kandel, E. (2012). *The age of insight*. New York: Random House.

Kandel, E. (2018). *The disordered mind*. New York: Farrar, Strauss & Giroux.

LeDoux, J. (2015). *Anxious*. New York: Viking.

McGilchrist, I. (2009). *The master and his emissary*. New Haven: Yale University Press.

Messer, S. (2001). Applying the visions of reality to a case of brief therapy. *Journal of Psychotherapy Integration*, 10, 55–70.

Messer, S. & Kaslow, N. (2020). Current issues in psychotherapy theory, practice, and research: A framework for comparative study, in S. Messer & N. Kaslow (Eds.), *Essential psychotherapies*, 4th edn (pp. 3–34). New York: Guilford Press.

Safran, J. & Messer, S. (1998). Barriers to psychotherapy integration, in J. Safran (Ed.), *Widening the scope of cognitive therapy* (pp. 269–293). Northvale, NJ: Jason Aronson.

Sapolsky, R. (2017). *Behave: The biology of humans at our best and worst*. New York: Penguin.

Schore, A. (2019a). *The development of the unconscious*. New York: Norton.

Schore, A. (2019b). *Right brain psychotherapy*. New York: Norton.

Siegel, D. (2020). *The developing mind*, 3rd edn. New York: Guilford.

Solms, M. (2018a). The scientific standing of psychoanalysis. *British Journal of Psychiatry International*, 15(1), 5–8.

Solms, M. (2018b). The neurobiological underpinnings of psychoanalytic theory and therapy. *Frontiers in Behavioral Neuroscience*. doi: doi:10.3389/fnbeh.2018.00294.

Strenger, C. (1997). Hedgehogs, foxes, and critical pluralism, *Psychoanalysis and Contemporary Thought*, 20 (1), 111.

Winnicott, D. W. (1945/1975). Primitive emotional development, in D. W. Winnicott, *Through paediatrics to psychoanalysis* (pp. 145–156). New York: Basic Books.

Part I
Pragmatism

Although the science of mind promises to deepen our understanding of the dynamics of behavior and theories of change across the foundational schools of psychotherapy, neither neuroscience nor theoretical formulations can tell us what particular actions will be therapeutic in the given clinical situation. This is why it is crucial to establish orienting perspectives, basic principles, and values that guide critical thinking and facilitate efforts to consider ideas and methods across the therapeutic traditions as we carry out our practice.

In Chapter 1 I explore fundamental elements of pragmatic philosophy and propose a working formulation of clinical pragmatism. I review concerns and themes that William James and John Dewey pursued in developing their classical versions of pragmatism and show how their contributions provide points of reference in our efforts to establish a working formulation of clinical pragmatism in therapeutic practice. I outline basic values and principles that guide our efforts to consider divergent ideas and methods across the schools of thought, bridging scientific and humanistic domains of understanding. In doing so I emphasize the individuality of the person and subjectivity; collaboration, open-ended dialogue, and the co-creation of meaning; the dynamics of experiential learning; and the practical outcomes of ideas and methods over the course of help and care. As we will see, the principles of clinical pragmatism help us join the findings of neuroscience and theories of psychotherapy with the phenomenal realm of the individual in the concrete particularity of the clinical situation.

1 Toward a Clinical Pragmatism

> Owing to the fact that all experience is a process, no point of view can ever be the last one.
>
> –William James

A diverse group of thinkers shaped the emergence of pragmatism at the end of the 19th century, creating what scholars have come to see as a distinctive American philosophy.[1] William James and John Dewey, the principal architects of classical pragmatism, emphasize pluralist approaches to understanding and the practical outcomes of beliefs and ideas in everyday life. James traces the term to the Greek word of the same name, meaning "action," from which our words "practice" and "practical" come (1907/1975, p. 28). Our theories should seek to serve human good, James argues, and the fundamental aim of knowledge ought to be concrete outcomes that help us negotiate the challenges of everyday living. The mind is ever active, experimenting, creating, adapting. In the most fundamental sense, as Louis Menand emphasizes, pragmatism is about "*how* we think, not what we think" (1997, p. xxvi). The approach is practical and instrumental, focused on immediate concerns, searching for what is useful, finding what works.

James, widely recognized as the leading American psychologist and philosopher at the turn of the 20th century, graduated from Harvard Medical School and became an academic celebrity following the publication of his classic work, *The Principles of psychology*, in 1890. Although he had hoped to establish psychology as a science of mind, he challenged the reductive materialism of the late 19th century, introducing versions of pluralism and pragmatism in his later writings on psychology and religion. Working as a phenomenologist, he sought to document the essence of the divine in *The Varieties of Religious Experience*, published in 1902, exploring the concrete realities of inner life, belief, and faith. In fashioning his pragmatic point of view, he emphasizes the plurality of factors that influence our experience and acknowledges the limits inherent in human understanding, urging us to approach concerns from multiple, independent perspectives, encompassing scientific and humanistic points of view.

He challenges any account of reality that would divorce it from the concrete particularities of actual experience. For James, the world of everyday life is "multitudinous beyond imagination, tangled, muddy, painful, and perplexed," continually presenting us with ambiguities and complexities, confusions and contradictions; the universe, in his rendering, is better understood as a "multi-verse" (1907/1975, pp. 17–18). Our paradigms of explanation offer but "a summary sketch, a picture of the world in abridgement, a foreshortened bird's eye view" of the immediacy and particularity of real life (1909/1967, p. 8).

In advancing his pluralist point of view, accordingly, James rejects conceptions of a unitary world of experience set forth in philosophical systems of monism and notions of grand theory, based on what we take to be objective, absolute truths. His pragmatism challenged the grand, sweeping visions of Kant, Hegel, and Schopenhauer. No single paradigm can encompass the multiplicity and complexity of human life, he argued; we can never synthesize our experience into a unified whole. At best our theoretical formulations offer but fragmentary, provisional renderings of experience.

James challenges us to consider different ways of seeing, understanding, and acting as we approach our work. There is room for novelty, contingency, and engagement of divergent ideas. We find equally valid points of view that inevitably contradict one another yet lead to insight, understanding, and action. Differing lines of inquiry may converge, providing a basis for belief—for our best guess as to the "truth" of the matter—but we are willing to accept the limits of our understanding, ever aware of the dangers of presuming to know too much. According to his notion of fallibilism, we regard uncertainty and contingency as conditions of knowledge. "The fundamental fact about experience is that it is a process of change... Owing to the fact that all experience is a process," he writes, "no point of view can ever be *the* last one" (1904/1975, p. 220–221).

For James, our ideas are tools for thinking and problem-solving. Theories, he explains, are "instruments, not answers to enigmas, in which we can rest. We don't lie back on them, we move forward... Pragmatism unstiffens all our theories, limbers them up and sets each one at work" (1907/1946, p. 53). In the pragmatic tradition, as Menand explains, an idea "has no greater metaphysical status than, say, a fork. When your fork proves inadequate to the task of eating soup, it makes little sense to argue about whether there is something inherent in the nature of forks or the something inherent in the nature of soup that accounts for the failure. You just reach for a spoon" (Menand, 2001, p. 361). Thinkers did not believe that ideas are "'out there' waiting to be discovered, but are tools—like forks and knives and microchips—that people devise to cope with the world in which they find themselves" (2001, xi). The question is what we can do with any particular idea—what concrete difference it makes in the particular and unreproducible circumstances of everyday living.

James was an empiricist before he became a pragmatist, as Dewey observes, and he came to think of pragmatism as empiricism carried to its conclusion (1925/1998, p. 7). The pragmatist rejects "abstraction," "absolutes," "fixed principles," and "closed systems," he writes, searching for "fact," "concreteness," "action," and "adequacy" in light of the practical tasks of the particular project, (James, 1907/1946, pp. 43–81). We can think of pragmatism as an open system, embracing the experience of ambiguity, complexity, and uncertainty, allowing the practitioner to join the unexpected and the odd. Richard Sennett characterizes James as a philosopher of "street smarts," explaining: "the maker follows a crooked path from the possible to the doable" (2018, p 9). In the most fundamental sense James believes that we should approach experience as "experiments in adapting to need," cautioning us not to equate the pragmatic with systematization, speed, or efficiency, ever attuned to the needs, possibilities, and constraints of the particular situation.

Action and experience, James shows in his accounts of pragmatism, serve as the final test of beliefs and ideas. In his view, truth *happens* to an idea: it is made real, becomes true, through the concrete particulars of experience. In following the pragmatic method, he writes, "You must bring out of each word its practical cash value, set it at work within the stream of your experience. It appears less a solution, then, than as a program for more work, and more particularly as an indication of the ways in which existing realities may be changed" (1907/1946, p. 53). The strength of the pragmatic approach, James emphasizes, lies not in beliefs or ideas but in the outcomes of experience.

James returns to the practical consequences of ideas in elaborating his pragmatic conceptions of truth: "The true is the name of whatever proves itself to be good in the way of belief and good, too, for definite, assignable reasons" (James 1907/1946, p. 76). If we take an idea to be true, he asks, "what concrete difference will its being true make in any one's actual life?… What, in short, is the truth's cash value in experiential terms?" (James, 1907/1946, p. 200). For James, the question is not "Is it true?" but rather "How would our lives be better if we were to believe it?" What is the use of a truth in any given situation?

Dewey, a public intellectual, political activist, and social reformer, drew on James' work in developing his accounts of pragmatism that would influence social, political, and cultural life through the 20th century. His scholarly work encompassed the disciplines of psychology and philosophy, but he is best known for his work in the field of education, where he is regarded as one of the most influential practitioners of the Socratic tradition. He joined the faculty of the University of Chicago in 1894, where he established the Laboratory School, an experiment in progressive education that continues to this day to emphasize the importance of active learning and engagement of practical concerns in everyday life. He worked closely with Jane Addams, participating in the programs of Hull House, and his writings informed progressive social, political, and industrial practices in the early 20th century. He brought a moral energy to his accounts of war and peace, race relations, women's suffrage, and economic alienation. His focus on the social surround and his faith in experimentation and action shaped distinctive visions of the emerging social work profession (Borden, 2013; Orcutt, 1990; Rockefeller, 1991).

In fashioning his pragmatism Dewey seeks to bridge the gap between thought and action, focusing on the particular contexts of experience and the ways in which we make use of intelligence to address real problems in everyday life. Action should be intelligent and reflective, guided by curiosity and open-minded, flexible, deliberative habits of thinking (1925/1998, p. 12). Like James, Dewey embraces pluralism, believing that multiple lines of inquiry strengthen understanding and action, and he centers on the practical consequences of beliefs and ideas in efforts to address "the active urgency of concrete situations" (1931, p. 219).

In elaborating his version of pragmatism, however, Dewey comes to emphasize the crucial role of collaborative interaction and experiential learning in our efforts to generate understanding and negotiate problems in living (Dewey, 1897/1998). He argues that philosophers have made a false distinction between knowing and doing, and he introduces the principle of *learning by doing*. In creating the Laboratory School he embraced the pedagogical functions of real activity in everyday life. Children would tend a garden, care for animals, cook, and weave cloth. He thinks of knowing and doing as indivisible features of the same process, active and muscular, fundamentally concerned with learning, adaptation, and instrumental outcomes. Our task is to raise questions, to figure things out, to act, to learn from experience. We learn by doing; we call upon the knowledge we have gained as we proceed with our work; the outcomes we generate continue to deepen and enlarge understanding, which we bring to bear in the next experience.

Experiential learning is an ongoing, self-corrective process; we clarify and revise our conceptions of knowledge in light of changing circumstance and outcomes. When we limit conceptions of knowledge to textbooks, Dewey argues, we deprive it from the authority of our lived experience and compromise our relations with the world. Knowledge is, in essence, "an instrument or organ of successful action" (Menand, 1997, p. xxiv).

He emphasizes the critical importance of context in his formulations of learning and understanding, emphasizing the dynamics of process and change: "We are not explicitly aware of the role of context just because our every utterance is so saturated with it that it forms the significance of what we say and hear" (Dewey, 1931, p. 204). We can think of "experience," Dewey writes, as "a process of undergoing: a process of standing something... Our undergoings are experiments in varying the course of events; our active tryings are trials and tests of ourselves" (1917/1998, p. 49).

Pragmatism and Therapeutic Practice

Although pragmatic sensibilities have shaped the course of therapeutic practice across the foundational schools of thought over the years, philosophically minded practitioners are rare, and there has been surprisingly little treatment of American pragmatism in the clinical literature. A series of writers have noted the absence of interest in pragmatic thought, proposing that it offers fundamental if largely unexamined principles and ethical perspectives for clinicians engaged in therapeutic practices (Borden, 1998, 1999; Brendel, 2006; Goldberg, 2002; Raposa, 2015; Strenger, 1997).

I first found myself speaking of a "clinical pragmatism" three decades ago in my seminar on Donald Winnicott and the Independent Tradition in British psychoanalysis, moved by unexpected points of connection with the work of James and Dewey. The Independent Tradition had emerged as a pragmatic voice in the 1940s, challenging the theoretical orthodoxy of Melanie Klein and Anna Freud. The clinicians who refused to embrace the purist paradigm of either thinker formed what is known as the "Middle Group," preserving an independence of mind, drawing on ideas and methods from divergent perspectives. Following the example of Winnicott, they were committed to a theoretical pluralism, emphasizing the ambiguities, complexities, and contingencies of the clinical situation, approaching their practice from multiple points of view without recourse to notions of absolute truth.

Like James and Dewey, they rejected objective or rational conceptions of knowledge, arguing that we can never know the truth of the whole, and they remained uneasy with sweeping assertions about personality, psychopathology, or the therapeutic endeavor, realizing the dangers of presuming to know too much. Their theoretical formulations originate in the concrete particulars of everyday practice, shaped by close observation and careful description of experience in accord with their empirical disposition. In line with James and Dewey, they emphasize the practical outcomes of ideas and methods, searching for what proves useful in the given case (see Borden, 1994, 1998, 2009; and Phillips, 1988, for expanded accounts of Winnicott and the Independent Tradition).

Carlo Strenger and Arnold Goldberg have offered valuable treatments of pragmatic philosophy and ethics in their writings on contemporary psychoanalysis and comparative psychotherapy.

Strenger explores the tension between purist approaches and pragmatism in his account, introducing a position he describes as "critical pluralism" (1997). In working from a purist point of view, Strenger argues, "the risk is that patients come to feel that they have been tied onto a Procrustean bed and cut or stretched to fit its size" (1997, p. 123). Although he does not engage American pragmatism, he draws on the pragmatic philosophy of John Stuart Mill and Isaiah Berlin in articulating a range of clinical and ethical concerns. Pragmatic thinkers reject "big ideologies and singlemindedness in the pursuit of One Truth" (p. 123) and embrace a "critical pluralism," realizing that "human understanding is intrinsically limited; that no conceptual framework can capture all possible perspectives on reality... and that the coexistence of competing conceptual frameworks is in itself of enormous value" (p. 128).

From a pragmatic perspective, Strenger explains, we do not deal with theory for theory's sake but "ultimately with a craft committed to helping people," rejecting purity of approach, relying on different ways of understanding, common sense, and flexibility as we search for what works. The defining feature of pragmatism, he writes, is our insistence that "the map must never be confused with the territory. It sees theory as a tool rather than as a mirror of reality, and hence judges its validity by its usefulness" (1997, p. 123).

Goldberg draws on James, Dewey, and Charles Sanders Peirce in his essay, presenting pragmatism as "a philosophy of instrumentalism or one devoted to the tools of a trade," regarding theory not as a rendering of objective knowledge about human behavior but as a tool for dealing with the complexities of clinical practice (2002, p. 236). He emphasizes the "effectiveness of diversity" in his discussion of theoretical pluralism and proposes that beneficial outcomes are more likely to follow from flexible use of ideas from divergent schools of thought rather than from a "final, unifying, overarching theory that puts it all together in a neat package" (p. 246). Only the test of effectiveness, he argues, should move us to choose one theory over another.

David Brendel, trained as a psychiatrist and philosopher, shows how pragmatic principles help clinicians negotiate fundamental tensions between science and humanism in his trenchant critique of psychiatry (2006). In the domain of science, clinicians draw on a range of heuristics, explanatory concepts, and empirical findings that carry the potential to deepen understanding of problems in functioning and inform treatment options. Yet reductive or rigid application of scientific research may restrict the range of help and care. Humanistic approaches focus on the person as an individual, taking account of the complexities of subjective experience, relational life, and existential concerns. The clinician must join scientific reasoning and humanistic values in efforts to care for the whole person, drawing on multiple perspectives that bridge both domains of understanding.

The pragmatic perspective he outlines in his book, informed by close readings of Peirce, James, and Dewey, is organized around what he calls the "four P's," emphasizing: 1) the practical dimensions of all scientific inquiry; 2) the pluralistic nature of the phenomena studied by science; 3) the participatory role of individuals with different perspectives in the social process of scientific inquiry; and 4) the provisional nature of scientific understanding and explanation (Brendel, 2006, p. 28). In his pragmatic approach, taking account of scientific reasoning and humanistic values, he challenges "the longstanding tendency to split the patient in to an objective specimen for scientific study," regarding the individual as a "complex human subject" whose experience evokes empathy, respect, compassion, and wonder (2006, p. 24).

Like Strenger and Goldberg, Brendel views the core ethical value of clinical pragmatism as "the primacy of practical results for individual persons in the everyday life world" (2006, p. 142). We do not think of beneficial outcomes "from an abstract or objective vantage point," he explains, "but rather in terms of the deliberations and negotiations among people working toward those goals" (2006, p. 142). I return to these accounts as we explore pragmatic conceptions of therapeutic action.

Clinical Pragmatism

Drawing on the classical thought of James and Dewey, I outline orienting perspectives, attitudes, values, and concerns that guide our efforts to establish a working formulation of clinical pragmatism in therapeutic practice. I explore the ways in which the core elements of pragmatic thought inform critical thinking and decision-making over the course of the therapeutic process, focusing our attention on crucial aspects of help and care, and show how the basic principles of pragmatism enlarge conceptions of therapeutic action and facilitating processes across the foundational schools of thought.

Individuality, Subjectivity, and the Human Particularity of the Therapeutic Process

In working from a pragmatic perspective, we focus on the individuality of the person. James centers on the realm of subjectivity, where he finds "a uniqueness that defies all formulation" (1911/1979, p. 109). When we engage "private and personal phenomena," he proposes, "...we deal with realities in the completest sense of the term" (1902/1985, p. 386). Above all, he emphasizes, our experience is *personal*: every sensation, feeling, image, thought, or action is mine or yours. "The only states of consciousness that we naturally deal with are found in personal consciousnesses, minds, selves, concrete particular I's and you's" (1893, p. 153). Dewey, emphasizing notions of personal agency, regards the individual as "the carrier of creative thought, the author of action, and of its application;" in his account, the "individual mind" is "the vehicle of experimental creation" (1925/1998, p. 12). James and Dewey both recognize the ways in which the changing contexts of experience influence what we see, hear, feel, think, and do, shaping the course of meaning and understanding.

Pragmatic values center our attention on the subjectivity of the individual, notions of personal agency and self-determination, and the unique circumstances of the clinical situation that defy categorization, deepening our appreciation of the complexities, ambiguities, and contingencies that inevitably shape the therapeutic process. The pragmatic perspective, accordingly, challenges a "technical rationalism" and reductive approaches to help and care based on rigid adherence to particular models of intervention, empirical findings, or technical procedures.

For example, although cognitive-behavioral therapy is widely regarded as the gold standard of treatment for post-traumatic stress disorder, other approaches have proven effective as well, including psychodynamic psychotherapy, humanistic and experiential forms of psychotherapy, hypnotherapy, mindfulness meditation, eye-movement desensitization and reprocessing, and yoga (Lambert, 2013; Wampold, 2010). In one of the largest studies of cognitive-behavioral treatment, Bessel Van der Kolk reported in his influential account of trauma, *The body keeps the score*, more than a third of the patients dropped out, and many suffered adverse reactions (Van der Kolk, 2014; also see Shedler, 2015). Different approaches prove more or less useful in light of the particular circumstances of the clinical situation as well as differences in personality and temperament, values and sensibilities, capacities and skills, and earlier experiences of help and care. We cannot know in advance what will prove to be "therapeutic" in light of the actual possibilities and constraints of the given case.

While standardized treatments focused on specific disorders and symptoms have their place in the broader landscape of clinical practice, pragmatic thinkers propose that effective outcomes depend largely on idiographic approaches based on our recognition and care of the whole person as an individual and the ways in which practitioners and patients make use of different elements in the clinical situation, rather than on nomothetic approaches that impose rigid models of intervention.

Although educators and scholars often frame psychotherapy as if it were a research-driven practice, guided by empirical study, protocols, and technical procedures, Brendel points out that "hard-nosed" and "inflexible diagnostic and therapeutic approaches"—even if researchers regard them as "evidence-based"— potentially harm patients, failing to take account of the range of conditions that influence capacities to make use of different approaches in the clinical situation (2006, p. 23; also see Messer & Kaslow, 2020; Shedler, 2015; Wampold, 2010). The principles and values of pragmatism help us justify and defend what we are willing (and unwilling) to say and do as we carry out our practice. I explore these concerns further in my accounts of clinical practice in Chapter 9.

Relationship, Collaboration, and Interactive Experience

Following Dewey's accounts of the crucial role of relationship and collaboration in our efforts to work toward understanding and action, pragmatic approaches reaffirm notions of egalitarianism and participation, emphasizing the fundamental importance of dialogue and an open-minded, deliberative process between the practitioner and the patient as they explore concerns. Clinical formulations are provisional, shaped by the patient's capacities to make use of different elements in the therapeutic process, experiential learning, and concrete outcomes over the course of care.

We continue to recalibrate our understanding of the authority of the practitioner and the patient in our conceptions of the therapeutic relationship, challenging views of the clinician as the all-knowing expert. Following developments across the foundational schools of thought explored in Part III, clinical scholars increasingly think of both parties as vulnerable, fallible, and capable, seeing the therapeutic endeavor as an active, searching process, facilitated through critical inquiry, dialogue, experiential learning, action, and reflection on outcomes (Berlin, 2005; Borden, 2013, 2014). The patient and the therapist bring their authority of experience to bear, revising their understanding of matters in light of ongoing outcomes. In accordance with the notion of fallibilism, we accept the limits of our understanding and remain open to experiential learning that deepens insight and informs action.

Researchers continue to document the crucial role of the quality of the relationship between the patient and the practitioner, the strength of the therapeutic alliance, and collaborative interaction in outcomes across the foundational schools of thought (Borden & Clark, 2012; Kazdin, 2007; Messer & Kaslow, 2020; Norcross & Wampold, 2018; Shedler, 2010; Wampold & Imel, 2015). We can trace the concept of the therapeutic alliance to Freud and the first generation of psychodynamic thinkers, but clinicians across the schools of thought have come to recognize it as a core condition of all forms of practice. Even therapists who embrace a technical eclecticism now regard the alliance as a necessary if not sufficient condition of change.

Researchers have emphasized three domains of concern in their formulations of the therapeutic alliance: the attachment bond between the patient and the therapist; mutual agreement on the goals of treatment, and shared understanding of the core activities of the therapeutic process (Horvath & Bedi, 2002). Following reformulations of therapeutic action in relational psychoanalysis, however, practitioners increasingly think of the alliance as an ongoing *process of negotiation* between the patient and clinician about tasks and goals, emphasizing the mutuality of the therapeutic process (Safran, 2012). The therapeutic alliance is the one of the most powerful predictors of therapeutic outcomes (Lambert, 2013, 2015; Messer & Kaslow, 2020; Norcross, 2011; Norcross & Wampold, 2018; Wampold & Imel, 2015).

As we will see, clinical scholars propose that the therapeutic relationship and the dynamics of interactive experience foster change in multiple ways. In the domain of interpersonal neurobiology, researchers believe that the core conditions of the therapeutic relationship engage biological mechanisms that enhance neuroplasticity. New and different ways of relating potentially alter networks of association in neural structures, including motives, emotions, and defensive processes linked to subjective states, representations of self and others, and behavior (Borden, 2009; Gabbard & Westen, 2003; Schore, 2019a, 2019b; Westen & Gabbard, 2002a, 2002b). The experience of attunement and synchrony in the interactive experience and the constancy of care in the holding environment, mediated by right-brain modes of communication, may strengthen internal functions instrumental in the regulation of emotion and subjective states (Borden, 2009; Schore, 2019a, 2019b). Ongoing interaction facilitates efforts to process and formulate experience, deepen capacities for reflection, and develop more functional patterns of behavior through the dynamics of internalization, modeling, and experiential learning. The working alliance serves as a catalyst, helping the patient more fully engage the core activities of the therapeutic process and make use of enriching relationships and activities in everyday life (see Wachtel, 2011).

Pluralist Orientation, Bridging Scientific and Humanistic Domains of Understanding

In accord with the pluralist orientation of pragmatic thought we recognize the value of scientific and humanistic realms of understanding, working to master a range of orienting perspectives, theories, therapeutic languages, models, and methods of intervention.

In the domain of science, emerging lines of study in the fields of genetics, neuroscience, evolutionary biology, and developmental psychology continue to strengthen our understanding of vulnerability, problems in living, and therapeutic practice. As a teacher and practitioner I follow developments in empirical research across diverse fields of study, trying to determine what is valid, sensible, and useful in light of the realities of everyday practice and the concrete particularities of the clinical situation. In accord with the values of pragmatic thought, however, we avoid rigid or reductive application of research findings, treatment guidelines, or protocols. In the following chapter we explore non-reductive versions of materialism that allow us to think of ourselves as physical beings without reducing mind and meaning to the dynamics of brain activity.

We rediscover the crucial importance of humanistic values at a time when renderings of help and care are shaped largely by a technical rationalism and reductive models of evidence-based practice. The humanities help us consider fundamental concerns in the clinical situation, enlarging ways of seeing, understanding, and acting. The liberal arts challenge the abstractions of theory and the generalizations of empirical research, enriching our faculties of reflection, imagination, emotion, and empathy, strengthening our capacities to negotiate the irreducible ambiguities, complexities, ironies, and inconsistencies of human experience.

The thinkers who shaped the emerging field of psychotherapy at the turn of the 20th century came to see the humanities as a foundation of clinical training, emphasizing the ways in which literature, mythology, and the arts deepen our appreciation of fundamental concerns in the human situation, challenging practitioners to consider questions of meaning and purpose, agency and will, freedom and justice, limitation and loss.

The sensibilities that we cultivate through our engagement of stories, novels, poetry, theater, art, music, and film deepen our capacities to negotiate the experience of difference, limits, vulnerability, and suffering as we carry out our practice, working to recognize and respect the individuality of the person. The humanities make a world worth living in, as the philosopher Martha Nussbaum observes, where we come to see other human beings as "full people, with thoughts and feelings of their own that deserve respect and empathy" (2010, p. 143). Robert Coles has documented the power of narrative in his moving accounts of adversity and misfortune, exploring the ways in which stories deepen our understanding of ourselves and the experience of others (1989, 1997, 2010). We come to appreciate the workings of fate, circumstance, and fortune that shape people and lives.

The foundational schools of psychotherapy differ in the philosophical perspectives, root metaphors, narratives, values, purposes, rules, models, and methods that shape training and practice. While we may think of a particular theory or model of practice as a "first language" or "home base," we do not privilege any single perspective over other approaches that would potentially help us address the practical needs of the individual in the given case. There is no single overarching theory. The pluralist perspective allows us to consider the ideas and methods of "purist" thinkers selectively in light of the needs of the clinical situation.

As I show in my accounts of clinical practice in Chapter 9, we may combine ideas and methods from divergent approaches that would be considered incompatible in more pure renderings of the therapeutic endeavor within the foundational schools of thought. From the perspective of clinical pragmatism, there is no single criterion or authorized method that can be used to determine the validity of a therapeutic construct; there is no universal measure of its success (Borden, 1994, 2009, 2010, 2014).

We assume that beneficial outcomes follow from attuned and flexible use of different ideas and methods across the schools of thought. In following a clinical pragmatism, as we will see, we think of psychotherapy as an *open practice* that is governed by our capacities to make use of different elements, experiential learning, and concrete outcomes rather than by fixed commitments to particular theoretical perspectives, empirical findings, or technical strategies per se. We realize that one approach may be more helpful than another at different points in the therapeutic process.

The therapeutic experience demands a richer vocabulary than any single theory or model can give it. Embracing the virtues of theoretical pluralism, Jerome Frank emphasizes the crucial functions of heuristics that provide plausible explanations of problems in living and the core activities believed to foster change and growth over the course of help and care. As we will see, the science of mind and the foundational schools of thought offer theories that help therapists and patients make sense of what is the matter and what carries the potential to help. They provide plausible explanations of problems in living and the ways in which core activities of the therapeutic process bring about change and growth. Cogent and coherent explanations of problems in living and the rationale of therapeutic activities strengthen morale, self-efficacy, and mastery (Frank & Frank, 1991; Wampold, 2010; Wampold & Imel, 2015). Although the dominant world views of particular cultures shape our perceptions of the authority and plausibility of different therapeutic rationales and practices, our notions of what makes sense are also influenced by personality and temperament, values and sensibilities, and earlier experiences of help and care; professional training, group identities, and institutional loyalties; reason and empirical evidence; and the possibilities and constraints of the clinical situation.

While no particular theory or heuristic appears to be empirically superior to any other, Frank emphasizes that the patient and the clinician must *believe in* the potential value of the approach they have taken. And, as Bruce Wampold points out in his discussion of common factors, there *is* empirical support documenting the crucial importance of our belief and faith in the efficacy and effectiveness of the theories and methods we engage over the course of the therapeutic process (Wampold, 2010, p. 110). Researchers continue to explore the neurophysiological processes that mediate the beneficial effects of belief, faith, and hope (for reviews of research on the magnitude of the placebo effect see Cozolino, 2017, and Sternberg, 2009).

Reflection-in-Action, Experiential Learning and Practical Outcomes

Following Dewey, we think of doing and knowing as indivisible aspects of the same process, and we call upon opportunities for experiential learning within the therapeutic process itself as well as in the relationships, activities, and surrounds of everyday life. We embrace pragmatic formulations of ideas as tools for thinking, drawing on different perspectives in light of changing needs, capacities to make use of various elements, and emerging concerns over the course of the therapeutic process. We carry out "experiments in adapting to need," moving from the possible to the workable, judging the validity of differing approaches in light of their "cash value."

Donald Schon, drawing on Dewey's notion of learning by doing, challenges conceptions of "technical rationality" that represent practitioners as instrumental problem-solvers who select technical means best suited to particular purposes on the basis of empirical findings (1983, 1987). He introduces the notion of "reflection-in-action" in his efforts to capture the dynamics of skilled practice, emphasizing the clinician's ongoing reflection and appraisal of evolving conditions and circumstances in a rapid, implicit, holistic fashion. In his account of professional excellence, the practitioner frames the "problematic situation," selecting particular concerns for attention, guided by an assessment of conditions and circumstances that brings coherence and direction for action; he describes it as an "ontological process"—"a form of worldmaking," in the phrase of Nelson Goodman (1978, p. 36).

In accord with Dewey's formulations of interpersonal collaboration, Schon reaffirms the crucial role of "reflective conversation" between the practitioner and the patient that facilitates revision of understanding and action in light of evolving outcomes. Following the idiographic perspective introduced earlier, we recognize the unique nature of the therapeutic process and realize the limits of systematic practices delivered in a standardized manner. Experiments in adapting to need take precedence over notions of efficiency. Above all, as Dewey observes, a pragmatic intelligence is a *"creative intelligence*, not a routine mechanic… intelligence frees action from a *mechanically instrumental character"* (1917, pp. 63–64, italics added). The clinician must consider a range of approaches in the search for what will be facilitative in the given moment.

As I have emphasized, the therapeutic process is guided by what proves useful rather than by fixed commitments to theoretical systems, empirical findings, or technical procedures. Pragmatism validates the authority of our experience. As Menand observes, it encourages us to trust our own judgments—to have faith that if we do what is right, the rest will follow (1997, xxxiv).

Psychotherapy Research and Clinical Pragmatism

Researchers have documented the efficacy and effectiveness of psychotherapy over the last half century, and we have come to think of therapeutic practices as powerful forms of help, care, and healing. As decades of studies show, the benefits of psychotherapy are considerable. Meta-analyses of outcome research demonstrate the effectiveness of treatments across a range of diagnostic conditions, populations, and settings.[2] A variety of approaches developed in the foundational schools of thought carry the potential to help patients reduce symptoms, reinstate healing processes, strengthen coping capacities, and improve interpersonal functioning. Patients deepen understanding and develop skills over the course of therapy that they continue to engage after treatment has ended, maintaining gains and strengthening capacities (for reviews and analysis of efficacy and effectiveness research see Kazdin, 2007; Lambert, 2013, 2015; Shedler, 2010, 2015; Solms, 2018; Wampold, 2010; Wampold & Imel, 2015).

We know that psychotherapy works. From the start of research on therapeutic practice, however, clinical scholars have differed in their beliefs about the particular factors thought to account for change and growth over the course of care.

In a seminal paper that pointed to the general equivalence of different approaches, published in 1936, Saul Rosenzweig proposed that all forms of psychotherapy share basic elements that account for their effectiveness. Beyond the particular beliefs and methods associated with different approaches, he argued, "there are inevitably certain unrecognized factors in any therapeutic situation" that may be "even more important than those being purposely employed" (Rosenzweig, 1936, p. 412). In his account of core elements he emphasized the crucial functions of the therapeutic relationship and the role of theoretical formulations that provide plausible explanations of problems in living and curative factors over the course of treatment. He called upon Lewis Carroll's Alice in Wonderland in his formulation of the dodo bird verdict: "At last the Dodo said, 'Everybody has won, and all must have prizes'" (1936, p. 412).

Jerome Frank drew on Rosenzweig's contributions in developing his conceptual framework for psychotherapy, focusing on the functions of the therapeutic relationship, the social and cultural contexts of healing practices, conceptual schemes that provide cogent explanations of problems and therapeutic interventions, and core activities that strengthen morale, mastery, capacities, and skills (Frank & Frank, 1991). According to the common factors perspective, we assume that therapeutic approaches exert their effects largely through core processes that operate independently of technical procedures associated with particular schools of thought.

Other researchers challenge this view, however, believing that we will come to identify specific factors that account for the relative effectiveness of particular approaches. The "specificity hypothesis" has guided efforts to establish a technical eclecticism in the domain of evidence-based practice. Briefly, the goal is to match specific methods of intervention with circumscribed problems in functioning on the basis of empirical findings and clinical knowledge. In a prescriptive version of this approach, clinicians use standardized treatment protocols linking diagnostic categories and technical procedures that they seek to validate in randomized controlled clinical trials.

We find some evidence that certain techniques are potentially more effective than others in the treatment of circumscribed symptoms, and some studies suggest that the beneficial effects of cognitive-behavioral approaches tend to decay over time. Overall, however, there is currently no convincing evidence that one approach is better than another for the wider range of problems in living that clinicians address in the day to day practice of psychotherapy (Lambert, 2013; Shedler, 2015; Wampold, 2010; Wampold & Imel, 2015). At this point, meta-analyses of research attempting to determine the relative efficacy of differing therapeutic approaches continue to show that all are roughly equally effective, supporting theory-driven approaches across the foundational schools of thought, documenting common effects across treatments. These findings challenge conceptions of psychotherapy that posit specific treatment effects for specific disorders, pointing to the crucial role of common factors and core activities rather than technical procedures in determining outcomes (Lambert, 2013; Norcross & Wampold, 2018; Shedler, 2015; Wampold, 2010; Wampold & Imel, 2015).

It is possible that unexamined assumptions and the nature of the methods that have shaped research thus far have limited our ability to determine whether significant differences do exist across different approaches, and continued study may yet document the strengths of particular models or techniques. Shedler speculates that the Dodo bird verdict may reflect a failure of investigators to consider the wider range of phenomena engaged over the course of the therapeutic process (2010).

Even so, the single-mechanism theories of therapeutic action set forth in purist models of practice fail to reflect the wider range of conditions and processes that are likely to account for the beneficial outcomes we find across divergent forms of treatment. Drawing on the orienting perspectives of neuroscience and the outcomes of psychotherapy research, it is reasonable to assume that change and growth occur through multiple mechanisms of therapeutic action, each of which may be engaged by different techniques.

In reformulating concepts of therapeutic action, clinical scholars reaffirm the fundamental role of core processes that are likely to be helpful for all patients as well as particular techniques that may be useful for some and not others. As Frank explains, the core activities of divergent forms of psychotherapy serve basic functions thought to foster change and growth. They challenge our experience of demoralization, helplessness, and hopelessness by strengthening the therapeutic relationship and collaborative alliance, creating expectations of help, offering new learning experiences, intensifying emotion, deepening a sense of efficacy and mastery, and generating opportunities for practice of new behaviors (Frank & Frank, 1991, p. 44). In light of our differing capacities to make use of particular approaches and methods, however, we realize that certain forms of therapeutic action may be more or less useful in the given case (see Chapter 9; also Borden, 1998, 2014; Gabbard & Westen, 2003; Kazdin, 2007).

In accordance with the principles and values of the pragmatic approach I have outlined here, the *ways* in which the therapeutic process is carried out are more important than the particular theoretical perspective, model of intervention, or technical procedure. As we have seen, pragmatic conceptions of help and care emphasize fundamental concerns that are likely to determine outcomes on the basis of the research evidence and clinical experience: the crucial importance of our focus on the person as an individual and subjective domains of experience; the core conditions of the therapeutic relationship, the collaborative alliance, open-ended dialogue, and the dynamics of interactive experience; pluralist approaches to understanding that offer plausible ways of formulating what is the matter and what carries the potential to help, strengthening a sense of hope and expectation; varied opportunities for experiential learning, fostering a sense of mastery and development of capacities and skills; and ongoing assessment of progress and outcomes over the course of treatment. The test for pragmatic knowledge is whether it effectively guides actions that bring about intended results in the given case.

We sometimes speak as if the question of what is therapeutic can be resolved by empirical research. It *is* an empirical question, but it is one that we can answer only in the concrete particularity of the given case. Our evaluations of therapeutic outcomes are shaped by differing concerns and problems in living, goals and expectations, values and worldviews. Life is not a controlled clinical trial, and we cannot know in advance how we will come to understand what is the matter or how we will make use of different elements over the course of the therapeutic experience. As Caro Strenger reminds us, we find ourselves working in a profession that will never be able to rely on algorithms to guide the ways we carry out our practice (1997, p. 144).

Notes

1 Louis Menand traces the origins of American pragmatism in *The Metaphysical Club* (2001), an intellectual history documenting the ways in which the first generation of thinkers, Charles Sanders Peirce, Oliver Wendell Holmes, James, and Dewey shaped the intellectual movement. For the purposes of this work I focus on the contributions of James and Dewey, the principal architects of classical pragmatism. See Gerald Meyers (1986) and Robert Richardson (2006) for intellectual biographies of James and critical analyses of texts; see W. R. B. Lewis (1991) for a study of the James family; see S. Rockefeller (1991) for an intellectual biography of Dewey. I expand earlier accounts of pragmatic philosophy and psychotherapy in this chapter (see Borden 1994, 1998, 2009, 2010, 2013, and 2014).

2 The first major meta-analysis of psychotherapy outcome research, published in 1980, included 475 studies and yielded an effect size of 0.85 for patients who received treatment compared with untreated control subjects (Smith, Glass & Miller, 1980). As Jonathan Shedler notes in his review of findings, an effect size of 0.80 is considered a large effect in psychological research (2010). Meta-analyses have continued to document comparable effect sizes, providing strong support for the efficacy of psychotherapy (for reviews of recent meta-analyses see Solms, 2018).

References

Berlin, S. (2005). The value of acceptance in social work direct practice: A historical and contemporary view. *Social Service Review*, 79(3), 482–510.

Borden, W. (1994). *Legacies of the independent tradition: Toward a clinical pragmatism.* Keynote address, Theory Matters Conference, 14 October, University of Chicago, Chicago, IL.

Borden, W. (1998). The play and place of theory in practice: A Winnicottian perspective. *Journal of Analytic Social Work*, 5 (1), 25–40.

Borden, W. (1999). Pluralism, pragmatism, and the therapeutic endeavor in brief psychodynamic psychotherapy, in W. Borden (Ed.), *Comparative approaches in brief dynamic psychotherapy* (pp. 7–43). New York: Haworth.

Borden, W. (2009). *Contemporary psychodynamic theory and practice.* New York: Oxford University Press.

Borden, W. (2010). Taking multiplicity seriously, in W. Borden (Ed.), *Reshaping theory in contemporary social work* (pp. 3–27). New York: Columbia University Press.

Borden, W. (2013). Experiments in adapting to need: Pragmatism as orienting perspective in clinical social work. *Journal of Social Work Practice*, 27 (3), 259–271.

Borden, W. (2014). Neuroscience, clinical pragmatism, and therapeutic action. Rhoda G Sarnatt Lecture, University of Chicago, Chicago, IL.

Borden, W. & Clark, J. (2012). Contemporary psychodynamic theory, research, and practice: Implications for evidence-based interventions, in T. Rzepnicki, S. McCracken & H. Briggs (Eds.), *From task centered social work to evidence-based and integrative practice* (pp. 65–87). New York: Oxford University Press.

Brendel, D. (2006). *Healing psychiatry: Bridging the science/humanism divide.* Cambridge: The MIT Press.

Coles, R. (1989). *The call of stories.* Boston: Houghton-Mifflin.

Coles, R. (1997). *Doing documentary work.* New York: Oxford University Press.

Coles, R. (2010). *Handing one another along.* New York: Random House.

Cozolino, L. (2017). *The neuroscience of psychotherapy* (3rd edn). New York: Norton.

Dewey, J. (1897/1998). My pedagogic creed, in L. Hickman & T. Alexander (Eds.), *The essential Dewey: Pragmatism, education, and democracy* (pp. 229–235). Bloomington, IN: Indiana University Press.

Dewey, J. (1917/1998). The need for a recovery of philosophy, in J. Dewey (Ed.), *Creative intelligence: Essays in the pragmatic attitude* (pp. 3–69). New York: Holt.

Dewey, J. (1925/1998). The development of American pragmatism, in L. Hickman & T. Alexander (Eds.), *The essential Dewey: Pragmatism, education, and democracy* (pp. 3–13). Bloomington, IN: Indiana University Press.

Dewey, J. (1931). Context and thought. *University of California Publications in Philosophy*, 12 (3), 203–224.

Frank, J. & Frank, J. (1991). *Persuasion and healing.* Baltimore: John Hopkins University Press.

Gabbard, G. & Westen, D. (2003). Rethinking therapeutic action. *International Journal of Psychoanalysis*, 84, 823–841.

Goldberg, A. (2002). American pragmatism and American psychoanalysis. *The Psychoanalytic Quarterly*, 71 (2), 235–250.

Goodman, N. (1978). *Ways of worldmaking.* Brighton, Sussex: The Harvester Press.

Horvath, A. & Bedi, R. P. (2002). The alliance, in J. N. Norcross (Ed.), *Psychotherapy relationships that work: Therapist contributions and responsiveness to patients* (pp. 37–69). New York: Oxford University Press.

James, W. (1893). *Psychology*. New York: Henry Holt.

James, W. (1902/1985). *The varieties of religious experience*. Cambridge, MA: Harvard University Press.

James, W. (1904/1975). Humanism and truth, in W. James (Ed.), *Pragmatism and the meaning of truth* (pp. 203–226). Cambridge, MA: Harvard University Press.

James, W. (1907/1946). *Pragmatism*. New York: Longmans, Green.

James, W. (1907/1975). *Pragmatism and the meaning of truth*. Cambridge, MA: Harvard University Press.

James, W. (1909/1967). *Essays in radical empiricism and a pluralistic universe*. Gloucester, MA: Pete Smith.

James, W. (1911/1979). *Some problems of philosophy*. Cambridge, MA: Harvard University Press.

Kazdin, A. (2007). Mediators and mechanisms of change in psychotherapy research. *Annual Review of Clinical Psychology*, 3, 1–27.

Lambert, M. J. (2013). The efficacy and effectiveness of psychotherapy, in M. J. Lambert (Ed.), *Bergin and Garfield's handbook of psychotherapy and behavior change*, 6th edn (pp. 169–218). New York: Wiley.

Lambert, M. J. (2015). Effectiveness of psychological treatment. *Resonanzen. E-Journal fur biopsychosoziele dialogue in psychotherapie, supervision und Beratung*, 3 (2), 87–100.

Lewis, R. W. B. (1991). *The Jameses: A family narrative*. New York: Farrar, Straus & Giroux.

Menand, L. (1997). *Pragmatism*. New York: Vintage.

Menand, L. (2001). *The metaphysical club*. New York: Farrar, Straus & Giroux.

Messer, S. & Kaslow, N. (2020). Current issues in psychotherapy theory, research, and practice, in S. Messer & N. Kaslow (Eds.), *Essential psychotherapies*, 4th edn (pp.3–32). New York: Guilford.

Meyers, G. E. (1986). *William James: His life and thought*. New Haven, CT: Yale University Press.

Norcross, J. (2011). *Psychotherapy relationships that work: Therapist contributions and responsiveness to patients*, 2nd edn, New York: Oxford University Press.

Norcross, J. & Wampold, B. (2018). A new therapy for each patient: Evidence based relationships and responsiveness. *Journal of Clinical Psychology*, 74, 1889–1906.

Nussbaum, M. (2010). *Not for profit: Why democracy needs the humanities*. Princeton, NJ: Princeton University Press.

Orcutt, B. (1990). *Science and inquiry in social work practice*. New York: Columbia University Press.

Phillips, A. (1988). *Winnicott*. Cambridge, MA: Harvard University Press.

Raposa, M. (2015). Remarks concerning the relevance of pragmatism for contemporary psychotherapy. Paper, European Pragmatism Conference II, 9–11 September, Paris.

Richardson, R. D. (2006). *William James*. Boston, MA: Houghton-Mifflin.

Rockefeller, S. (1991). *John Dewey: Religious faith and democratic humanism*. New York: Columbia University Press.

Rosenzweig, S. (1936). Some implicit common factors in diverse methods of psychotherapy. *American Journal of Orthopsychiatry*, 6, 412–415.

Safran J. (2012). *Psychoanalysis and psychoanalytic therapies.* Washington, DC: American Psychological Association.

Schon, D. (1983). *The reflective practitioner.* New York: Basic.

Schon, D. (1987). *Educating the reflective practitioner.* San Francisco, CA: Jossey Bass.

Schore, A. (2019a). *The development of the unconscious mind.* New York: Norton.

Schore, A. (2019b). *Right brain psychotherapy.* New York: Norton.

Sennett, R. (2018). *Ethics for the city: Building and dwelling.* New York: Farrar, Straus & Giroux.

Shedler, J. (2010). The efficacy of psychotherapy. *American Psychologist,* 65 (2), 98–109.

Shedler, J. (2015). Where is the evidence for evidence-based therapy? *Journal of Psychological Therapies in Primary Care,* 4, 47–59.

Smith, M. L., Glass, G. V. & Miller, T. I. (1980). *The benefits of psychotherapy.* Baltimore, MD: Johns Hopkins University Press.

Solms, M. (2018). The neurobiological underpinnings of psychoanalytic theory and therapy. *Frontiers in Behavioral Neuroscience,* 12, 294.

Sternberg, E. (2009). *Healing spaces: The science of place and well-being.* Cambridge, MA: Harvard University Press.

Strenger, C. (1997). Hedgehogs, foxes, and critical pluralism: The clinician's yearning for unified conceptions. *Psychoanalysis and Contemporary Thought,* 20 (1), 111–145.

Van der Kolk, B. (2014). *The body keeps the score: Brain, mind, and body in the healing of trauma.* New York: Penguin.

Wachtel, P. (2011). *Inside the session.* Washington, DC: American Psychological Association.

Wampold, B. (2010). *The basics of psychotherapy.* Washington, DC: The American Psychological Association.

Wampold, B. & Imel, Z. (2015). *The great psychotherapy debate: The evidence for what makes psychotherapy work,* 2nd edn. New York and London: Routledge.

Westen, D. & Gabbard, G. (2002a). Developments in cognitive neuroscience: Conflict, compromise, and connectionism. *Journal of the American Psychoanalytic Association,* 50, 53–90.

Westen, D. & Gabbard, G. (2002b). Developments in cognitive neuroscience: Implications for theories of transference. *Journal of the American Psychoanalytic Association,* 50, 99–134.

Part II

The Science of Mind

William James and John Dewey prefigure our current understanding of neuroplasticity in their formulations of experiential learning, growth, and adaptation, believing that the expansion of experience fosters the development of the brain throughout life. Some scholars speak of the pragmatic philosophers as America's first cognitive neuroscientists, rediscovering the ways in which their conceptions of experience, learning, knowledge, and relational life anticipate fundamental developments in the science of mind.[1]

The fields of neuroscience continue to enlarge our understanding of growth and resilience across the course of life. Researchers have come to appreciate the role of nature and nurture in development, and we continue to discover the ways in which genetic action and experiential opportunities in the social surround shape the maturation of the brain and mind. We increasingly recognize the properties of neuroplasticity and the crucial role of relational life and experiential learning in the ongoing growth and integration of neural networks thought to underlie resilience, health, and well-being. The structure and function of the brain, shaped by experiential opportunities in the social surround, is unique to each individual. Conceptual syntheses bridging findings in the fields of genetics, evolutionary biology, neuroscience, cognitive psychology, developmental psychology, and cultural anthropology promise to strengthen our understanding of therapeutic action across the foundational schools of thought in contemporary psychotherapy.

I explore the implications of recent work in the science of mind for clinical practice in the second part of the book, showing how orienting perspectives deepen our understanding of therapeutic action in accord with the principles and values of clinical pragmatism. I begin Chapter 2 with a brief account of recent treatments of brain and mind in the philosophy of science and show how the pluralist orientation and the humanistic values of pragmatic thought allow us to think of ourselves as physical, mental, and relational beings without recourse to a reductive materialism, bridging biological, psychological, and social realms of experience. Although educators have increasingly realized the relevance of neuroscientific research for therapeutic practice, many clinical training programs fail to address the biology of mind in their curricula. In the following section I outline our current understanding of the dynamics of neural development and describe the core structures and functions of the brain. Finally, I review conceptual syntheses and empirical findings in the field of interpersonal neurobiology that carry particular relevance for psychotherapy, expanding our understanding of the dynamics of attachment and basic forms of memory.

In Chapter 3 I explore recent developments in our understanding of neuroplasticity and describe domains of neural integration that shape concepts of therapeutic action in the field of interpersonal neurobiology, drawing on the preceding overview of the brain. I introduce working hypotheses about the ways in which the core activities and processes of psychotherapy facilitate change and growth in light of the dynamics of brain function. While we must regard these proposals as partial and provisional, they offer points of reference in ongoing efforts to bridge the domains of neuroscience and psychotherapy, helping us consider the "cash value" of ideas and research findings.

The overviews in Part II provide orienting perspectives as we consider concepts of therapeutic action in Part III, exploring points of connection between neuroscience and the ways in which the facilitating processes and experiential learning of psychotherapy are thought to foster change and growth. As we will see, emerging lines of study in the science of mind reaffirm the crucial role of theoretical pluralism and diverse forms of therapeutic action in accord with the basic principles of clinical pragmatism.

Note

1 John Shook and Tibor Solymosi characterize pragmatism as a perennial philosophy "precisely because its core views on experience, cognition, learning, knowledge, values, psychological and education development, interpersonal relationships, and social organization enjoy regular confirmation by evolutionary biology, developmental psychology, experimental sociology, and the brain sciences including recent developments in neuroscience" (Shook & Solymosi, 2014, p. 1).

Reference

Shook, J. & Solymosi, T. (2014). *Pragmatist neurophilosophy: American philosophy and the brain*. London: Bloomsbury.

2   Orienting Perspectives in Neuroscience

...living creatures, first and last, have selves...

–Oliver Sacks

Contemporary philosophers of science continue to explore fundamental questions about the nature of mind and body—whether we think of the mental and the physical as one and the same or whether we regard the mind as a non-physical phenomenon independent of the body. Over the last century researchers in neurology and the fields of neuroscience have documented the close connections between the dynamics of brain function and patterns of sensation, emotion, thought, and behavior, challenging the notion of the disembodied mind that Descartes had proposed in his dualism. A series of clinical scholars, notably Kurt Goldstein, A. R. Luria, Antonio Damasio, and Oliver Sacks, have provided compelling accounts of cases drawn from their research and practice, exploring the ways in which brain pathology may bring about radical changes in personality and behavior, precipitating a range of problems in functioning (see, for example, Damasio, 1994; Goldstein, 1940, 1942; Luria, 1966, 1987; Sacks 1985, 1995, 2010, 2012). Most thinkers have come to embrace an ontological materialism, believing that we cannot conceive of the mind as a non-physical entity distinct from the brain. Even so, divergent points of view have shaped debate in the philosophy of neuroscience over the years, challenging clinicians to adopt a critical pluralism in their understandings of brain and mind as they carry out everyday practice.

Following the turn toward reductive biological models of explanation at the end of the 20th century, preceded by the "decade of the brain" in the 1990s, some thinkers predicted that psychological domains of understanding would recede in light of the growing power of neuroscience to account for the origins of problems in functioning and mechanisms of change and growth. Paul Churchland, Patricia Churchland, and Stephen Stich advanced positions in the philosophy of mind known as eliminative materialism, anticipating a time when psychological explanations of behavior would be replaced by scientific understanding across the fields of particle physics, atomic and molecular theory, organic chemistry, evolutionary biology, and neurophysiology (P.M. Churchland, 1981, 1995; P. S. Churchland, 1986). They proposed that mental states are fully reducible to the physical states of the brain, arguing that what we think of as mind or psyche has neither autonomy nor any causal power of its own, believing that biology would one day provide a unified explanation of human behavior (see P. S. Churchland, 2013). In a completed neuroscience, they predicted, we would come to see mental concepts as relics of an outdated psychology.

Other philosophers have challenged the reduction of mind and meaning to the neural, emphasizing the inherent gap between the observable dynamics of brain activity and the unobservable experience of subjectivity, consciousness, and the essence of the self. In his classic essay, "What is it like to be a bat?," Thomas Nagel argued that while our appreciation of neurophysiology allows us to understand the mechanisms of the sonar system—bats do not see but navigate through their sense of hearing and electromagnetic waves—it will never help us know "what it is like for a *bat* to be a bat" (1974, p. 439). He pointed to the gap between physical and phenomenological domains of experience in subsequent critiques of reductive materialism, arguing that consciousness has a subjective character, a *what it is like* feature, that the physical sciences alone cannot explain (Nagel, 2000).

David Chalmers has brought a muscular challenge to the materialist paradigm over the last quarter century, proposing that there is no property of the brain that can account for human subjectivity (Chalmers 1995, 1996, 2010, 2012). He argues that the subjective aspects of mental phenomena—ineffable qualities called *qualia*—are beyond the reach of human understanding. The nature of our subjective experience is fundamentally different from our understanding of the neurophysiology of the brain. Our experience of color, sound, smell, and touch—the look and feel and sense of things, the textures of life— cannot be reduced to the language of neurophysiology. My experience of the warm, rich red of the peonies I rediscovered every summer in my grandmother's garden cannot be explained by our understanding of the dynamics of activation in region V4 of the visual cortex. "Living creatures, first and last, have selves," Sacks reminds us in his accounts of brain and mind (1984, p. 177). Human reality is constituted by subjectivity. "What it is to be a person is shaped by what it is *like* for that person to be," Jonathan Lear writes. "The meanings, emotions, and desires alive in a person's soul play a crucial role in determining who that person is" (1990, p. 4).

William James and John Dewey criticized psychologists for treating mental states as if they were fixed, static properties of brain function. They viewed mind as *activity*, emphasizing dynamic processes of interaction. James describes the ways in which "psychic" as well as "physical" factors influence the operation of neural structures and functions. Consider, for example, the following passage from the *Principles of psychology*: "I hope that the reader will take no umbrage at my so mixing the physical and the mental, and talking of reflex acts and hemispheres and reminiscences in the same breath, as if they were homogeneous quantities and factors of one causal chain. I have done so deliberately; for although I admit that from the radically physical point of view it is easy to conceive of the chain of events amongst the cells and fibers as complete in itself, and that whilst so conceiving it one need make no mention of ideas, I yet suspect that point of view of being an unreal abstraction. Reflexes in centers may take place even where accompanying feelings or ideas guide them" (James, 1890/1945, p. 33).

James introduced the metaphor of the "stream of consciousness" to represent our ever changing experience of sensation, emotion, thought, imagery, and behavior. In doing so, as Richard Sennett notes, he challenged us to explore the ways in which the concrete particulars of place, relational life, and activity influence ongoing states of mind and body—"where you are, who is with you, what you or they are doing when you have a particular thought, feeling or sensation" (2018, p. 175).

Dewey expanded James' conception of consciousness in *Experience and nature*, elaborating a language of dynamic processes, emphasizing the ways in which changing contexts influence "a series of heres and nows" (1925, p. 230). "To see the organism *in* nature, the nervous system in the organism, the brain in the nervous system, the cortex in the brain is the answer to the problems which haunt philosophy. And when thus seen they will be seen to be *in*, not as marbles are in a box but as events are in history, in a moving, growing, never finished process" (1929, p. 241). Although there would be no mind without the brain, James and Dewey realized, we cannot reduce our understanding of all mental phenomena to brain states. The physical, the psychological, the social, and the environmental interact in complex ways. Neurobiological processes influence mental life and behavior, just as psychological and social processes influence physiological functions and bodily states.

The crucial question we must ask ourselves as practitioners, David Brendel emphasizes in his treatment of the mind-body problem, "is whether ontological materialists are justified in formulating explanations of human behavior that employ concepts from disciplines other than the physical sciences, such as psychology" (2006, p. 85).

Although research across the fields of neuroscience promises to deepen our understanding of the dynamics of brain activity, Brendel acknowledges it will never help us appreciate what it is like for us to be ourselves from the first-person perspective of lived experience, nor will it necessarily inform the ways we engage particular methods of help and care over the course of our therapeutic practices. He welcomes the advances of neuroscience, embracing a scientific outlook, but he rejects reductive versions of materialism that would foreclose humanistic paradigms of understanding. Drawing on the work of the philosopher Terence Horgan (1993), Brendel proposes "nonreductive materialism" as an alternative position. In following a non-reductive materialism, we assume that the psychological is ontologically part of the material world, but that mental properties exert causal influence without being reducible to physical properties (see Baker, 2009, for expanded account of nonreductive materialism).

The nature of human experience and the practical concerns of clinical practice require a multitude of explanatory concepts bridging scientific and humanistic domains of understanding. In accord with the principles of clinical pragmatism, as Brendel shows in his account, a non-reductive materialism allows us to draw on biological, psychological, and social perspectives in our efforts to understand the whole person as an individual, explain problems in living, and formulate different approaches to help and care in light of the givens of the clinical situation. The ideas and methods that we engage at any particular point are determined by the conditions, concerns, tasks, and outcomes of our practice rather than by fixed commitments to particular scientific or philosophical positions. In working from clinical pragmatism, we accept the proposal that while the efficacy of psychotherapy may lie largely in the ways the experience alters the structures and functions of the brain, we realize the need to move beyond the domains of neurobiology and consider a wider range of heuristics in our formulations of what it means to be human, what is the matter, and what carries the potential to help. In this sense, as Brendel explains, we think of psychotherapy as a pragmatic project rooted in ontological materialism and brain science (2006, p. 88).

As we consider the dynamics of change and growth in psychotherapy from the perspective of neuroscience, it is important to clarify the ways in which we are using the terms "brain" and "mind." For the purposes of our discussion, in accord with the non-reductive materialism outlined here, I draw on working definitions proposed by Daniel Siegel that shape understanding in the field of interpersonal neurobiology. He uses the term "brain" to refer to the extended nervous system, describing it as the "embodied neural mechanism that shapes the flow of energy and information," "intimately interwoven with the physiology of the body as a whole." (Siegel, 2020, p. 502). His conception of "mind" encompasses the domains of subjective experience; awareness; information processing; and a regulatory function that he describes as "an emergent, self-organizing, embodied, and relational process of the extended nervous system and relationships" (2020, p. 507). From this perspective we regard the activity of the brain as a fundamental part of mind. As he emphasizes, however, our conception of mind is "broader than the brain and bigger than the individual body. Mind is fully embodied and fully relational" (2020, p. 507). The orienting perspectives of interpersonal neurobiology, synthesizing concepts and empirical findings across a range of disciplines over the last two decades, guide the following accounts of neural development and the dynamics of brain function.

The Brain

The brain encompasses features of organization and function that have moved neuroscientists to call it "the most complicated material object in the known universe" (Edelman, 2004, p. 14). In spite of the rapid advances in the science of mind over the last three decades, our knowledge of neural processes remains surprisingly limited, and researchers continue to explore the organization, development, and functioning of the brain.[1]

We can trace our understanding of the basic structures and functions of the brain to the scientific and artistic gifts of Santiago Ramon y Cajal, the Spanish neuroanatomist. Toward the end of the 19th century he created techniques in microscopy that allowed him to document the structure and connections of the cells of the nervous system. He was one of the first researchers to study the cellular functioning of the brain, and scholars have come to think of him as the architect of modern neuroscience. He produced nearly 3,000 drawings over the course of his research—recognized as works of art in their own right, sometimes compared to the scientific illustrations of Leonardo da Vinci—that scholars regard both as observations and arguments about the dynamics of brain function (King & Himmel, 2017; for further accounts of his scientific and artistic contributions see Dubinsky, 2017; Swanson, 2017).

Cajal proposed that the brain is made up of discrete cells, known as neurons, rather than a continuous network of cell appendages, as most neuroanatomists at the time believed. Over the course of his work he introduced basic principles that have come to provide the conceptual foundations for our understanding of the brain and the nervous system. In his formulation of the Neural Doctrine, he proposed that the neuron is the basic structural and functional unit of the nervous system. He described the defining features of the neuron in his iconic drawings, detailing the dendritic spine that receives signals from other neurons, and the growth cone, the appendage that allows neurons to make synaptic connections with other neurons. In the Theory of Dynamic Polarization, he argued that information flows through nerve cells in one direction, moving from dendrites to cell bodies to axons.

In line with the thinking of Freud and James, Cajal elaborated conceptions of neuroplasticity, proposing that the brain continues to mature across the course of life. Drawing on the language of nature to describe the structures and functions of the brain, he compared the cerebral cortex "to a garden filled with innumerable trees, the pyramidal cells, which can multiply their branches thanks to intelligent cultivation, sending their roots deeper and producing more exquisite flowers and fruits every day" (Cajal, 1894, cited in Ferreira, Nogueira & DeFelipe, 2014, p. 1). He emphasized the ways in which experience changes the brain, and he recommended "cerebral gymnastics" for the ongoing development of mental functions, prefiguring our current practices of brain fitness (Ehrlich, 2017; see Ferreira, Nogueira & DeFelipe, 2014, for an account of the intellectual traditions and research that shaped Cajal's conceptions of neuroplasticity).

Dynamics of Neural Development

Neuroscientists estimate that the brain is made up of more than 80 billion neurons and trillions of glial cells that produce myelin and regulate the flow of blood, supporting the function of neural systems. As the working cell of the nervous system, the neuron receives and sends signals through electrical impulses and chemical transmissions, creating energy flows throughout the brain, forming complex circuits. As Cajal detailed in his drawings, the neuron consists of a cell body; receiving ends known as dendrites that resemble dense thickets, and long, sinuous, tubular fibers called axons that form connections with other neurons. In accord with his theory of dynamic polarization, the neuron sends an electrical impulse down the axon. Subsequent research showed that neurotransmitters are released at the synapse, which either activate or inhibit the adjoining neuron. The synapse serves as the point of contact in a border area between neurons, connecting them to one another. Researchers believe that each neuron makes between one thousand and ten thousand connections with other neurons (Kandel, Schwartz, Jessell, Siegelbaum & Hudspeth, 2013).

Patterns of activation create synaptic connections that organize the structures and functions of neural networks. As Donald Hebb explains in his classic axiom, neurons that fire together become "associated" so that "activity in the one facilitates activity in the other" (1949, pp. 69–70). In this sense we can think of the architecture of the brain as associational, as Freud and James had proposed toward the end of the 19th century. Freud functionally linked the activity of nerve cells early in his career as a neuroanatomist (Sulloway, 1979). James introduced "the law of association" in his account of brain function and the mind in the *Principles of psychology* (1890). When processes are stimulated jointly or immediately after one another, they proposed, the stimulus activates subsequent processes in a sequential order.

Experience shapes particular patterns of neuronal firing, and the dynamics of activation create distinctive configurations of sensation, emotion, cognition, imagery, and behavior that mediate states of self. What we register as "my experience," accordingly, corresponds to specific forms of neural activation. James thought of consciousness as a process, not a thing.

We understand "instantiations" as distinct patterns of neural activity that form a functional whole (Cozolino, 2017; Siegel, 2020). Experiential conditions activate particular patterns of firing. My grandmother cared for me as a child, and we gardened together every morning through the spring and summer. More than half a century later, the scent of lilacs, the yellow of forsythia, the feel of damp earth, or the song of cardinals evoke the sense of her soothing voice and the encircling arms that held me. My experience of nature, relationship, and care was structured as neural networks—"instantiations"— that shape ongoing reactions and states of mind.

Experiential opportunities continue to reorganize the configurations of neural networks across the course of life, influencing states of mind and behavior, challenging earlier conceptions of the brain as fixed, programmed like a computer. The process by which experience brings about structural change in neural connections, known as Hebbian learning or long-term potentiation, is thought to be instrumental in neuroplasticity. We explore these concepts further in our review of neuroplasticity in the following chapter.

Basic Structures and Functions

Neurons and glia form structures within the brain, ranging from smaller networks known as nuclei to more complex systems described as circuits, regions, and hemispheres. More broadly, neuroanatomists distinguish three global areas of the brain, described as the lower region of the brainstem, which regulates fundamental physiological functions; the middle region of the limbic system, which mediates our experience of emotion and memory; and the upper region of the cerebral cortex, which controls perception, attention, thinking, and reasoning; these areas correspond to the "bottom," "middle," and "top" levels of the brain, following the hierarchical model of neural organization proposed by John Hughlings Jackson, the British neurologist, at the end of the 19th century.

   Although the nuclei, circuits, regions, and hemispheres serve different types of processing functions, generating distinct forms of knowledge and understanding, they are closely linked and form a functional system. The brain is highly interconnected, and specialized areas interact with hundreds of other regions. Charles Sherrington, one of the founders of neurophysiology, a colleague and lifelong friend of Cajal, imagined the awakening brain as "an enchanted loom where millions of flashing shuttles weave a dissolving pattern, always a meaningful pattern though never an abiding one; a shifting harmony of subpatterns" (1943, p. 178). Oliver Sacks offered a musical analogy, comparing the ongoing integration of regions to "something like a vastly complicated orchestra with thousands of instruments, an orchestra that conducts itself, with an ever-changing score and repertory" (2010, p. 104). Shortly after the turn of the century researchers introduced the term "connectome" to represent the structural and functional interconnections believed to shape global states of brain function; neuroscientists describe the oscillation of neural firing in waves of energy patterns that link different regions into a functional whole as "connectome harmonics" (see Siegel, 2020, for expanded accounts of neural integration and the connectome).

The Lower Region

The brain stem, located at the bottom of the brain, regulates fundamental physiological processes, including temperature, respiration, reflexes, heart rate, and blood pressure. From an evolutionary perspective it is the oldest structure of the brain, often called the reptilian brain, and we can think of it as the neural substrate of the somatic realm of experience. Hughlings Jackson characterized this region as the physiological bottom of the mind (1931).

   The autonomic nervous system governs states of alertness and arousal and the dynamics of the fight, flight, or freeze response. High levels of arousal activate the sympathetic network, releasing adrenalin, preparing us for fight or flight. The parasympathetic network activates the release of acetycholine, lowering lowers levels of arousal, promoting self-preservative functions. Drawing on the work of Charles Darwin, Steven Porges has explored the ways in which the double-branched cranial nerve known as the vagus, connecting the brain with the heart, lungs, stomach, and intestines, governs our reactions to threat (2011). When we register danger, we instinctively attempt to engage others, searching for help, support, and reassurance. If others fail to respond the "vagal brake" is released, mobilizing the sympathetic branch, preparing us for fight or flight. If the threat is acute, the more primitive dorsal vagal system is activated, leading to the immobilization of "freeze" or "collapse" reactions. We can think of the dissociative states that follow trauma as the psychological complement to this physical state. As we restore a sense of safety, the myelinated ventral vagus activates the "vagal brake" that slows the sympathetic nervous system, calming the body, restoring equilibrium (see Van der Kolk, 2014, for expanded account of polyvagal theory and trauma).

The lower portion of the brain contains the hypothalamus and the pituitary, which regulate physiological homeostasis through neuronal firing and hormonal release. Researchers continue to explore the complex interactions between the lower brain functions and other systems of the body, advancing our understanding of the ways in which the autonomic nervous system and the neuroimmune system mediate states of self, attachment and relational life, reactions to stress and trauma, and illness experience (see Cacioppo, Cacioppo, Capitanio & Cole, 2015; McEwen, 2008; Sapolsky 2017; Schore, 2019a, 2019b; Siegel, 2020; Sternberg, 2001, 2009).

The body-sensing regions of the lower structures of the brain create neural representations of somatic states thought to influence feelings, thoughts, and behaviors. Antonio Damasio has explored the relationships between the body, mind, and emotion in his pioneering studies of homeostasis, subjectivity, and the experience of the self, deepening our understanding of the role of subcortical and cortical structures in mapping somatic states in the brain (Damasio, 1994, 1999, 2010, 2018; Damasio & Caravalho, 2013).

Drawing on the work of William James, he proposes that the core of self-awareness is closely linked to physical sensations originating in the brain stem that register our experience of the body through signals from organs, tissues, muscles, and the joints of the skeleton. Body and mind are inseparable. We experience our sense of aliveness through "somatic markers" and primordial feelings—"wordless, unadorned, and connected to nothing but sheer existence" (Damasio, 2010, p. 21). The making of the mind and the creation of feeling is mediated by the interaction of the nervous system and the rest of the body (see Damasio, 2018, for an expanded account of homeostasis, mind, subjectivity, and culture; see parallels with the depth psychology of C. G. Jung in Chapter 4).

The Middle Region

The limbic structures of the brain, encompassing the amygdala and the hippocampus, lie between the brain stem and the cerebral cortex. The neural networks of this area regulate sources of arousal in the brain stem and higher-level processing in the cerebral cortex, integrating basic mental processes, playing a major role in our experience of perception and attention, the activation of emotion, and the appraisal of meaning, learning, and memory. This region evolved with the emergence of mammals, and it is instrumental in the establishment of the attachment bond that facilitates caretaking and relational life; it is thought to underlie our sense of a "unitary self" (Markowitz & Stanilou, 2011).

The connectivity of the amygdala system allows it to link distant regions throughout the brain, influencing global states of functioning. Under conditions of threat, the amygdala signals the brainstem to activate the sympathetic nervous system that mediates the fight or flight reaction. Although accounts of the brain often describe the amygdala as the "fear center," it is responsive to positive experience as well, generating a range of emotional reactions (see Todd & Anderson, 2009, for expanded account of the adaptive functions of the amygdala system). As we will see shortly, the amygdala matures before the hippocampus, and it is instrumental in the formation of implicit memory, registering early experience as unconscious, pre-symbolic emotional memories that exert a global and disproportionate influence on the dynamics of sensation, emotion, cognition, and behavior (LeDoux, 2015; Sapolsky, 2017). The hippocampus begins to mediate the organization of explicit memory and conscious processing of life events in the second year of life, allowing us to place our experience in context and time as we develop capacities for autobiographical memory.

The Upper Region

The cerebral cortex, the "top" part of the brain, is the last structure to develop and it continues to mature across the course of life through ongoing experience, activity, and learning. From an evolutionary perspective it is the most recent structure, sometimes called the neo-mammalian brain. This region guides our efforts to process information and carry out the activities of everyday life, governing the executive functions of the brain, mediating capacities for perception, self-awareness, regulation of emotion, focused attention, thought, reasoning, judgment, decision-making, problem-solving, planning, and strategic action (for an expanded review of the structures and functions of the upper region see Cozolino, 2017; Sapolsky, 2017; and Siegel, 2020).

Over the course of evolution the two halves of the cerebral cortex have come to serve different functions. Recent studies of brain laterality continue to document fundamental differences between the right and left hemispheres. Though the regions are closely linked through the corpus callosum, they differ in their organization and modes of processing experience, moving some researchers to speak of a "conscious left brain system" and an "unconscious right brain system" (Schore, 2019b).

Iain McGilchrist reviews the history of brain laterality research in his pioneering work, *The master and his emissary*, concluding that the right and left hemispheres create radically different versions of the world, shaping divergent ways of attending to experience as we negotiate and synthesize opposing realities (2009). In the realm of the right hemisphere, he proposes in a recent essay, we experience "the live, complex, embodied world of individual, always unique, beings, forever in flux, a net of interdependencies, forming and reforming wholes…" (2019, p. 22). In the domain of the left hemisphere, we experience what he describes as a "re-presented" version of our experience, containing "static, separable bounded, but essential fragmented entities, grouped into classes on which predictions can be based. This kind of attention isolates, fixes, and makes each thing explicit by bringing it under the spotlight of attention…" (2019, p. 22). In developing his formulations he emphasizes: "These are not different ways of *thinking about* the world: they are different ways of *being in* the world" (2019, p. 22).

Researchers distinguish a "left-brain surface, verbal, conscious, analytical explicit self" and a "right-brain deeper, nonverbal, nonconscious, holistic, emotional, corporeal, subjective implicit self" (Schore, 2019b, p. 185). The left hemisphere, associated with capacities for logic, linearity, literal thinking, and language, is thought to be instrumental in sequential processing, focused attention, and top-down processing of experience (Rogers, 2014; Schore, 2019b). The right hemisphere is central in processing emotion and nonverbal, holistic, visuospatial domains of experience; the region is closely linked with empathic functions, modulation of stress, and integrated maps of the whole body, dominant in bottom-up systems that regulate states of self.

As McGilchrist explains, the right hemisphere helps us see things in their uniqueness, embedded in the concrete particularities of the real world, while the left hemisphere, given to abstraction and reduction, helps us classify and categorize things (2019). He points to research findings supporting the primacy of the dynamics of the unconscious and emotion over conscious will, proposing: "The right hemisphere both grounds our experience of the world at the bottom end, so to speak, and makes sense of it, at the top end" (2015, p. 100; for an expanded review and discussion of research on bilaterality see Cozolino, 2017; Schore, 2019a, 2019b; and Siegel, 2020). We explore the functions of each hemisphere further in our discussion of horizontal integration in Chapter 3.

The two hemispheres of the cerebral cortex are divided into four lobes, named after the bones that cover them. By way of overview, the frontal lobes govern executive functions, moral reasoning, regulation of emotion, and movement. The parietal lobes connect sensory experience and motor functions with vision, hearing, and balance, creating an embodied sense of self in the world. The right parietal lobe plays a central role in helping us create spatial maps and mental models of the world—our relationship to people, objects, and threats within our immediate surrounds. The left parietal lobe is closely linked with capacities for abstraction, word-finding, metaphor, and arithmetic. The occipital lobes regulate our visual processing of experience and contain distinct areas specialized for different aspects of vision, such as form, color, and motion. The temporal lobes mediate higher perceptual functions, including auditory processing, receptive language, and memory functions. The upper part of the left temporal lobe contains a region known as Wernicke's area that mediates the comprehension of meaning and the semantic aspects of language. Each lobe serves distinct functions, though there is considerable interaction among them (for expanded accounts see Kandel, 2012; Ramachandran, 2011; and Siegel, 2020).

The prefrontal cortex encompasses two systems, broadly described as the dorsolateral prefrontal cortex and the orbitomedial prefrontal cortex. The systems differ in their biochemistry, architecture, connectivity, and functions (see Cozolino, 2017, for an expanded review).

The dorsolateral region, the conscious realm of the rational mind, is specialized for cognitive intelligence. The networks of this area are closely linked with the hippocampus and the left hemisphere, instrumental in our efforts to focus attention, process experience, formulate our understanding of circumstances, reason, problem-solve, and plan. Robert Sapolsky describes the dorsolateral region as "the decider of deciders," the most utilitarian part of the prefrontal cortex (2017).

The structures of the orbitoprefrontal cortex, closely linked to the amygdala and right hemisphere, mediate the dynamics of attachment, subjective experience, emotional regulation, and communication. The networks of this system are thought to play a central role in interoception, self-awareness, and mentalization, influencing the ways in which we perceive and interpret the feelings, thoughts, and intentions of others (Fonagy, Gergely, Jurist & Target, 2002). Clinical scholars continue to explore the ways in which the structures and functions of this area influence the dynamics of attachment, relational life, and therapeutic action (see Schore, 2019a, 2019b; Siegel, 2020; Wallin, 2007). The middle prefrontal systems integrate divergent structures of the brain, balancing the cortical activity of cognition with sensory and emotional experience through the lower regions of the brain and body proper (Cozolino, 2017; Damasio, 2018; Schore, 2019b; Siegel 2020).

Neural circuits process and synthesize our experience of sensation, emotion, imagery, cognition, and behavior, mediating states of self and functional outcomes. In optimal functioning, as discussed earlier, we assume that energy and information flow in multiple directions throughout the brain. As Damasio writes:

> Mind and behavior are moment-to-moment results of the operation of galaxies of nuclei and cortical parcels articulated by convergent and divergent neural projections. If the galaxies are well-organized and work harmoniously, the owner makes poetry. If not, madness ensues.
>
> (2010, p. 312)

Attachment and Brain Development

Conceptual syntheses and empirical study in developmental psychology continue to bridge the fields of neuroscience and psychotherapy. From the perspective of interpersonal neurobiology, as Allan Schore has shown in his integrations of theory, research, and clinical experience, we think of the attachment relationship as the major organizer of brain development. The attachment bond, the dynamics of caretaking experience, and the course of relational life in the social surrounds of infancy and childhood are fundamental in shaping the architecture of the brain, mediating the development of integrative and regulatory functions. Ongoing attunement and patterns of synchrony in interaction and communication between the child and caregivers create neural networks, forming the core structures of the brain, integrating sensory, emotional, cognitive, and behavioral domains of experience.

Over the course of his work Schore has increasingly centered on emotion and the dynamics of unconscious processes in his reformulations of classical attachment theory, shifting the focus from patterns of overt behavior that shaped John Bowlby's original accounts of the attachment bond to the realm of intersubjectivity, communication, and interactive regulation between the child and caretakers (Schore, 2012, 2019a, 2019b).

The dynamics of synchrony, rupture, and interactive repair shape his reformulations of attachment. By way of overview, the more the caregiver contingently tunes levels of activity to the infant during periods of social engagement, the more the caregiver allows the infant to recover quietly in periods of disengagement, and the more the caregiver attends to the infant's initiating cues for reengagement, the more synchronized their interaction. Following lapses in attunement and rupture, the caretaker re-regulates negative states and restores synchrony.

In the ongoing dialogue, he proposes, the caretaker and the infant co-construct cycles of "affect synchrony" that up-regulate positive emotion (joy, elation, excitement, interest) and "rupture and repair" that down-regulate negative emotion (fear, sadness, shame, disgust). The regulatory processes of emotional synchrony, which create states of positive arousal, and interactive repair, which modulates states of negative arousal, are the fundamental elements of attachment. The ongoing dynamics of attunement, rupture, and re-attunement in the relational matrix mediate the development of the emotion-processing limbic circuits of the right hemisphere, shaping the emerging self over critical periods of maturation in the first two years of life (Schore, 2012, 2019a, 2019b).

The right hemisphere is instrumental in the development of capacities for implicit relational knowing, the "nonconscious reception, expression, and communication of emotion and the cognitive and physiological components of emotional processing" (Schore, 2009, p. 6). A growing body of research supports the crucial functions of the right hemisphere in sense of self and relational life, mediating capacities for self-awareness, empathy, and identification with others (Decety & Chaminade, 2003; Knox, 2011; McGilchrist, 2019; Schore, 2019a, 2019b).

Donald Winnicott describes the experience of embodiment, aliveness, authenticity, creativity, and play in his accounts of the true self that emerges in the constancy of care over the course of infancy and childhood. Caregivers continue to shape the emerging self in formative ways. As David Wallin explains:

> The expressions of the child's self that evoke the attachment figure's attuned responsiveness can be integrated, while those that evoke dismissing, unpredictable, or frightening responses (or no responses at all) will be defensively excluded or distorted. What is integrated can then enjoy a healthy maturational trajectory; what is not tends to remain undeveloped... the difficulties that bring patients to treatment usually involve unintegrated and underdeveloped capacities to feel, think and relate to others (and to themselves) in ways that "work."
>
> (2007, p. 100)

Researchers assume that epigenetic programming by variations in the quality of caretaking strengthens resilience or increases risk for psychopathology and physical illness in adulthood and later life (Sroufe, 2016; Sroufe, Coffino & Carlson, 2010; Stevenson, Halliday, Marden & Mason, 2008). A large body of empirical findings shows that neglect, abuse, and trauma in infancy and early childhood increase risk for a range of conditions, including post-traumatic stress disorder, borderline personality disorder, and major depression (Roth, 2017; Roth & Sweatt, 2011; Schore, 2019a, 2019b; Siegel, 2020; Wallin, 2007; Van der Kolk, 2014). Adverse childhood experiences are linked with a range of negative health outcomes in adulthood, including diabetes, hypertension, heart disease, stroke, cancer, and dementia (see Dube, Felitti, Dong, Giles & Anda, 2003 for a review of the findings from the landmark Adverse Childhood Experience study).

Adversity compromises the regulatory functions of the body, influencing the course of synaptic growth, gene expression, and reactions to stress. "If children grow up with dominant experiences of separation, distress, fear, and rage," D. F. Watt writes, "then they will go down a bad pathogenic developmental pathway, and it's not just a bad psychological pathway but a bad neurological pathway" (2003, p. 109, cited in Schore, 2019b, p. 24).

We have come to think of our experience of attachment as an ongoing *process* rather than a fixed property, evolving across the course of development as we negotiate the dynamics of relational life. In accord with current understandings of neuroplasticity, we assume that the core conditions of the therapeutic relationship and enriching forms of experiential learning over the course of treatment carry the potential to reinstate developmental processes that have been compromised in earlier caretaking, reorganizing the deeper neural structures that mediate attachment, strengthening capacities to process and integrate subjective experience, regulate emotion, and negotiate the dynamics of relational life. As Schore and Wallin emphasize in their accounts, we can think of the integration of the core structures and functions of the brain as the neural corollary to the psychological integration we foster over the course of psychotherapy, connecting the body, states of mind, and behavior.

Memory

"If our view of memory is correct," Gerald Edelman and Giulio Tononi proposed at the turn of the century, "…every act of perception is, to some degree, an act of creation, and every act of memory is, to some degree, an act of imagination" (2000, p. 101). Over the last half century converging lines of study in the fields of cognitive psychology and neuroscience have documented two domains of memory, most broadly categorized as implicit and explicit. Researchers describe fundamental differences in the maturation, architecture, and dynamics of these forms of memory, and findings promise to deepen our understanding of vulnerability, problems in functioning, and basic tasks in psychotherapy.

We can trace the origins of modern memory research to the work of Brenda Milner, a British neuropsychologist who began her studies of cognition and learning at the Montreal Neurological Institute in the 1950s. In her case study of Henry Molaison, known as H.M., published in 1957, she described his profound loss of memory following an experimental surgical procedure intended to control his intractable epileptic seizures. After the removal of the medial temporal lobe, which contains the hippocampus, Molaison developed a pervasive loss of memory for people, places, and objects. His perceptual and intellectual functions remained intact.

In the course of her research, Milner found that Molaison was able to learn new motor skills though repetition, even though he was not conscious of the skills he was developing. He had lost his capacity for explicit memory—memory of people, places, and objects, based on conscious recall, dependent on the medial temporal lobe and the hippocampus. Yet he had preserved his capacity for implicit memory—the unconscious recall of motor skills, perceptual skills, and emotional experience, dependent on the amygdala. Milner's research documented the crucial role of the hippocampus in memory, showing that memory is a distinct set of mental functions located in particular structures of the brain. In time, researchers would demonstrate that memory is not a unitary faculty of mind (Milner, Squire & Kandel, 1998; Sacks, 2017).

Implicit Memory

Over the first year of life we register our experience as unconscious, pre-symbolic memories in the amygdala. The structures of implicit memory, functional before birth, organize unconscious patterns of learning across sensory, motor, and emotional networks as associative memories, encoded in layers of neural processing out of awareness.

When implicit memories are activated, the "instantiations" engage circuits in the brain that mediate fundamental aspects of experience in everyday life—the sensations, emotions, images, thoughts, and behaviors that constitute our sense of self, our perceptions of relational life, and our assumptive world—what we think of as "me," "my experience," "my world." In this sense we can think of our early states of mind as implicit forms of memory that influence the organization of the self and the development of traits that we understand as defining features of personality. Researchers assume that implicit memories shape the development of attachment schemas and working models of relational life that influence patterns of interpersonal behavior. Implicit memory operates in the experience of "priming," where contextual cues activate particular features of earlier experience in preparation for action (Schore, 2019a; Siegel, 2020; Van der Kolk, 2014).

The content of implicit memory, accordingly, is carried in our experience of sensations, emotions, perceptions, thoughts, and behaviors that remain unintegrated and unformulated, operating out of awareness. We do not experience the subjective sense of remembering in the realm of implicit memory; we feel, imagine, think, and act without any awareness of the influence of past events on present experience, not having access to the associative processes that underlie our experience. The effects of earlier events are present, here and now, without any sense of conscious memory (Westen & Gabbard, 2002 p. 68; see Siegel, 2020, for expanded accounts of memory).

We can think of patterns of attachment, transference reactions, defensive processes, and fundamental attitudes toward the self, others, and the world that originate in early states of mind as forms of implicit memory. A fundamental task of psychotherapy is to deepen understanding of the ways in which early experiences have shaped implicit memories that perpetuate problems in functioning.

Explicit Memory

The structures of explicit memory organize conscious forms of learning that require focal attention, reflected in recall of facts, ideas, and episodes. Endel Tulving, a cognitive neuroscientist and experimental psychologist at the University of Toronto, has advanced our understanding of explicit memory over the course of his research. He first made the distinction between memory of factual information and memory of personal experience in a report published in 1972, coming to classify explicit memory as semantic (referring to general knowledge of facts) or as episodic (referring to memory for specific episodes in time or autobiographical events) (Tulving, 2013).

As the medial temporal lobe matures in the second year of life we develop capacities for explicit memory, allowing us to register our experience of relational life, place, and time, organizing information according to context and sequence. In contrast to implicit memory, we can formulate our experience of learning, rendering it into words, fostering the development of autobiographical narratives and knowledge of self. The hippocampus plays a central role in the organization of explicit memory, as Milner had shown in her accounts of Henry Molaison.

The functional relationship between the amygdala and the hippocampus is thought to be a crucial determinant of top-down and right-left forms of neural integration, as we will see in the following chapter, influencing our capacities for perception, emotional regulation and learning. The amygdala is closely linked to "right" and "down" systems that govern somatic and emotional experience, while the hippocampus is instrumental in "left" and "top" systems that mediate conscious awareness and capacities to formulate and reflect on experience (Cozolino, 2017; Siegel, 2020).

Researchers assume that implicit memories of trauma carried in the networks of the amygdala and the right hemisphere potentially precipitate a range of problems in functioning. Bessel Van der Kolk provides a careful discussion of research documenting the ways in which recollections of emotional events from the past can activate the visceral sensations associated with the original event, disrupting basic bodily functions (2014). The experience of acute and prolonged stress generates the release of glucocorticoids thought to compromise the functioning of the hippocampus, leading to atrophy and memory deficits (Davidson & McEwen, 2012). Patients with post-traumatic stress disorder secondary to childhood trauma or combat exposure, chronic depression, and schizophrenia show hippocampal cell loss correlated with memory deficits (Cozolino 2017; Siegel, 2020; Van der Kolk, 2014). Louis Cozolino proposes that compromise in hippocampal functioning may increase the role of the amygdala in mediating memory, emotion, and behavior.

From the perspective of neuroscience, the therapeutic process carries the potential to strengthen the integration of networks linking unconscious and conscious domains of memory, helping patients bring implicit memories into awareness as they render experience into words, taking account of earlier events in reshaping narrative accounts of their lives. In psychodynamic concepts of therapeutic action, associative methods and processing of interactive experience in the therapeutic relationship are thought to engage the realm of implicit memory, helping patients reorganize unconscious associational networks that precipitate emotional reactions, defensive behavior, and patterns of interpersonal behavior that perpetuate problems in living. A range of approaches and techniques across the foundational schools of thought help patients engage and reorganize conscious patterns of feeling, thought, and behavior operating in the domain of explicit memory.

Note

1 Interdisciplinary research conducted in the 1990s, designated as "The decade of brain" by the National Institute of Mental Health and the Library of Congress, has shaped ongoing efforts to deepen our understanding of the biological mechanisms underlying mental processes. At the time of writing scientists are carrying out a collaborative effort known as the Human Connectome Project, modeled after the Human Genome Project, conceived by the National Institutes of Health and the National Science Foundation in the United States. Researchers seek to record the activity of every neuron in real time, linking the physical processes of the brain to the mental processes of the mind.

For expanded accounts of neuroanatomy, neural development, and the science of mind see Kandel, Schwartz, Jessell, Siegelbaum & Hudspeth (2013); for a comprehensive introduction to interpersonal neurobiology, synthesizing concepts and empirical findings across a range of scientific disciplines, see Siegel (2020).

References

Baker, L. (2009). Non-reductive materialism, in A. Beckermann, B. McLaughlin & S. Walter (Eds.), *Handbook of philosophy of mind* (pp. 109–120). New York: Oxford University Press.

Brendel, D. (2006). *Healing psychiatry: Bridging the science/humanism divide.* Cambridge, MA: MIT University Press.

Cacioppo, J., Cacioppo, S., Capitanio, J. P. & Cole, S. W. (2015). The neuroendocrinology of social isolation. *Annual Review of Psychology*, 66, 733–767.

Cajal, S. R. (1894. Consideraciones generales sobre la morfologia de la celula nerviosa. *La Veterinaria Espanola*, 37, 257–260, 273–275, 289–291.

Chalmers, D. (1995). Facing up to the hard problem of consciousness. *Journal of Consciousness Studies*, 2 (3), 200–219.

Chalmers, D. (1996). *The conscious mind: In search of a fundamental theory.* New York and London: Oxford University Press. Chalmers, D. (2010). *The character of consciousness.* New York: Oxford University Press.

Chalmers, D. (2012). *Constructing the world.* New York: Oxford University Press.

Churchland, P. M. (1981). Eliminative materialism and propositional attitudes. *Journal of Philosophy*, 78, 67–90.

Churchland, P. M. (1995). *The engine of reason, the seat of the soul: A philosophical journey into the brain.* Cambridge, MA: MIT Press.

Churchland, P. S. (1986). *Neurophilosophy: Toward a unified science of the mind-brain.* Cambridge, MA: MIT Press.

Churchland, P. S. (2013). *Touching a nerve: Our brains, our selves.* New York: Norton.

Cozolino, L. (2017). *The neuroscience of psychotherapy.* 3rd edn. New York: Norton.

Damasio, A. (1994). *Descartes' error: Emotion, reason, and the human brain.* New York: Putnam.

Damasio, A. (1999). *The feeling of what happens.* New York: Harcourt Brace.

Damasio, A. (2010). *Self comes to mind: Constructing the conscious brain.* New York: Pantheon/Random House.

Damasio, A. (2018). *The strange order of things.* New York: Pantheon.

Damasio & Caravalho, G. (2013). The nature of feelings: Evolutionary and neurobiological origins. *Nature reviews neuroscience*, 14 (2), 143.

Davidson, R. & McEwen, B. (2012). Social influences on neuroplasticity: Stress and interventions to promote well-being. *Nature Neuroscience*, 15 (5), 689–695.

Decety, J. & Chaminade, T. (2003). When the self represents the other: A new cognitive neuroscience view on psychological identification. *Consciousness and cognition*, 12 (4), 577–596.

Dewey, J. (1925). *Experience and nature.* Chicago, IL: Open Court.

Dewey, J. (1929). *The quest for certainty.* New York: Minton, Balch.

Dube, S. R., Felitti, V. J., Dong, M.Giles, W. H. & Anda, R. A. (2003). The impact of adverse childhood experiences on health problems: Evidence from four birth cohorts dating back to 1900. *Preventative Medicine*, 37 (3), 268–277.

Dubinsky, J. (2017). Seeing the beautiful brain today, in L. W. Swanson, E. Newman, A. Araque and J. M. Dubinsky (Eds.), *The beautiful brain* (pp. 193–202). New York: Abrams.

Edelman, G. (2004). *Wider than the sky: The phenomenological gift of consciousness.* New Haven, CT: Yale University Press.

Edelman, G. & Tononi, G. A. (2000). *A universe of consciousness: How matter becomes imagination*. New York: Basic Books.

Ehrlich, B. (2017). The hundred trillion stories in our head. *Paris Review Blog*, March 27.

Ferreira, R. M., Nogueira, M. I. & DeFelipe, J. (2014). The influence of James and Darwin on Cajal and his research into th neuron theory and the evolution of the nervous system. *Frontiers in Neuroanatomy*, 8, 1.

Fonagy, P., Gergely, G., Jurist, E. & Target, M. (2002). *Affect regulation, mentalization, and the development of the self*. London: Karnac.

Goldstein, K. (1940). *Human nature in the light of psychopathology*. Cambridge, MA: Harvard University Press.

Goldstein, K. (1942). *After effects of brain injuries in war*. New York: Grune & Stratton.

Hebb, D. O. (1949). *The organization of behavior: A neuropsychological theory*. New York: Wiley.

Horgan, T. (1993). Nonreductive materialism and the explanatory autonomy of psychology, in S. J. Warner & R. Warner (Eds.), *Naturalism: A critical appraisal* (pp. 295–320). Notre Dame, IN: University of Notre Dame Press.

Jackson, J. H. (1931). *Selected writings of John Hughlings Jackson*, Vols. 1 and 2. London: Hodder & Stoughton.

James, W. (1890/1945). *Principles of psychology*. London: Macmillan.

Kandel, E. H. (2012). *The age of insight*. New York: Farrar, Straus & Giroux.

Kandel, E. H., Schwartz, J. H., Jessell, T. M., Siegelbaum, S. A. & Hudspeth A. J. (2013). *Principles of neuroscience*, 5th edn. New York: McGraw Hill.

King, L. & Himmel, E. (2017). Drawing the beautiful brain, in L. W. Swanson, E. Newman, A. Araque and J. M. Dubinsky (Eds.), *The beautiful brain* (pp. 21–32). New York: Abrams.

Knox, J. (2011). *Self-agency in psychotherapy*. New York: Norton.

Lear, J. (1990). *Love and its place in nature*. New Haven, CT: Yale University Press.

LeDoux, J. (2015). *Anxious*. New York: Viking.

Luria, A. R. (1966). *Human brain and psychological process*. New York: Harper & Row.

Luria, A. R. (1987). *The man with a shattered world: The history of a brain wound* (L. Solotaroff, Trans.). Cambridge, MA: Harvard University Press.

Markowitz, H. J. & Stanilou, A. (2011). Amygdala in action: Relaying biological and social significance to autobiographical memory. *Neuropsychologia*, 49, 718–833.

McEwen, B. S. (2008). Central effects of stress hormones in health and disease: Understanding the protective and damaging effects of stress and stress mediators. *European Journal of Pharmacology*, 583 (2–3), 174–185.

McGilchrist, I. (2009). *The master and his emissary*. New Haven, CT: Yale University Press.

McGilchrist, I. (2015). Divine understanding and the divided brain, in J. Clausen & N. Levy (Eds.), *Handbook of neuroethics*. Dordrecht: Springer Science.

McGilchrist, I. (2019). *Ways of attending*. London and New York: Routledge.

Milner, B., Squire, L. & Kandel, E. (1998). Cognitive neuroscience and the study of memory, *Neuron*, 20, 445–468.

Nagel, T. (1974). What is it like to be a bat? *Philosophical Review*, 83(4), 435–450.

Nagel, T. (2000). *Mortal minds*. Cambridge: Cambridge University Press.

Porges, S. (2011). *The polyvagal theory: Neurophysiological foundations of emotion, attachment, communication, and self-regulation*. New York: Norton.

Ramachandran, V. (2011). *A brief tour of human consciousness*. New York: PI Press.

Rogers, L. (2014). Asymmetry of brain and behavior in animals: Its development, function, and human relevance. *Genesis*, 52, 555–571.

Roth, T.L. (2017). Epigenetic advances in behavioral and brain sciences have relevance for public policy. *Policy Insights from the Behavioral and Brain Sciences*, 4 (2), 202–209.

Roth, T. L. & Sweatt, J. D. (2011). Annual research review: Epigenetic mechanisms and environmental shaping of the brain during sensitive periods of development. *Journal of Child Psychology and Psychiatry*, 52 (4), 398–408.

Sacks, O. (1984). *A leg to stand on*. New York: Touchstone.

Sacks, O. (1985). *The man who mistook his wife for a hat*. New York: Simon & Schuster.

Sacks, O. (1995). *An anthropologist on Mars*. New York: Knopf.

Sacks, O. (2010). *The mind's eye*. New York: Knopf.

Sacks, O. (2012). *Hallucinations*. New York: Knopf.

Sacks, O. (2017). *The river of consciousness*. New York: Knopf.

Sapolsky, R. (2017). *Behave*. New York: Penguin.

Schore, A. (2012). *The science of the art of psychotherapy*. New York: Norton.

Schore, A. (2019a). *The development of the unconscious mind*. New York: Norton.

Schore, A. (2019b). *Right brain psychotherapy*. New York: Norton.

Sennett, R. (2018) *Ethics for the city: Building and dwelling*. New York: Farrar, Straus & Giroux.

Sherrington, C. S. (1943). *Man on his nature*. Cambridge: Cambridge University Press.

Siegel, D. (2020). *The developing mind*, 3rd edn. New York: Guilford.

Sroufe, L. A. (2016). The place of attachment in development, in J. Cassidy & P. R. Shaver (Eds.), *Handbook of attachment: Theory, research, and clinical applications*, 3rd edn (pp. 997–1011). New York: Guilford.

Sroufe, L.A., Coffino, B. & Carlson, E. A. (2010). Conceptualizing the role of early experience: Lessons from the Minnesota Longitudinal Study. *Developmental Review*, 30 (1), 36–51.

Sternberg, E. (2001). *The balance within*. New York: Freeman.

Sternberg, E. (2009). *Healing spaces: The science of place and well being*. Cambridge, MA: Harvard University Press.

Stevenson, C. W., Halliday, D., Marsden, C. & Mason, R. (2008). Early life programming of hemispheric lateralization and synchronization in the adult medial prefrontal cortex. *Neuroscience*, 155, 852–863.

Sulloway, F. (1979). *Freud: Biologist of the mind*. New York: Basic.

Swanson, L. (2017). Santiago Ramon y Cajal, in L. W. Swanson, E. Newman, A. Araque and J. M. Dubinsky (Eds.), *The beautiful brain* (pp. 11–21). New York: Abrams.

Todd, R. M. & Anderson, A. K. (2009). Six degrees of separation: The amygdala regulates social behavior and perception. *Nature Neuroscience*, 12, 1217–1218.

Tulving, E. (2013). *Memory, consciousness, and the brain: The Tallinn Conference*. Philadelphia, PA: Psychology Press.

Van der Kolk, B. (2014). *The body keeps the score: Brain, mind, and body in the healing of trauma*. New York: Penguin.

Wallin, D. (2007). *Attachment and psychotherapy*. New York: Guilford.

Watt, D. F. (2003). Psychotherapy in an age of neuroscience, in J. Corrigal & H. Wilkinson (Eds.), *Revolutionary connections: Psychotherapy and neuroscience* (pp. 79–115). London: Karnac.

Westen, D. & Gabbard, G. (2002). Developments in cognitive neuroscience: 1. Conflict, compromise, and connectionism. *Journal of the American Psychoanalytic Association*, 50, 53–98.

3 Neuroscience and Therapeutic Action

> The characteristic of the maturational process is the drive towards integration.
> –Donald Winnicott

Donald Winnicott writes powerfully of the "maturational process" and the fundamental "drive towards integration" that shapes the emergence of the self, emphasizing the crucial importance of "going on being" and "psyche-soma integration" in his formulations of development, health, and well-being (1963/1965, p. 239). Working as a pediatrician and psychoanalyst, he defined the "true self" as "the inherited potential which is experiencing a continuity of being and acquiring in its own way and at its own speed a personal psychic reality and a personal body scheme" (1960/1965, p. 46), originating in the experience of aliveness itself. From the perspective of neuroscience, as we have seen, the establishment of the self and the experience of well-being and resilience are closely linked to the integration of neural networks connecting the core structures of the brain. Daniel Siegel, the principal architect of interpersonal neurobiology, has come to think of integration as *the* fundamental mechanism of resilience, health, and optimal living, instrumental in the organization and regulation of the self, subjectivity, consciousness, and patterns of behavior.

In line with the working definition he has proposed, I use the term integration to describe the dynamics of basic processes that unify the systems of the brain and mind, regulating physiological homeostasis, emotion, sense of self, awareness, and adaptive functioning (Siegel, 2020). Researchers assume that energy and information flow in multiple directions throughout the brain in states of integration as neural circuits process and synthesize our ongoing experience of sensation, emotion, imagery, cognition, and behavior (Cozolino, 2017; Pribram, 1991).

A range of conditions potentially compromise the development and functioning of the brain, including genetic action, lapses in empathic attunement and responsiveness in caretaking, restrictions of opportunity, and various forms of traumatic experience. In the domain of interpersonal neurobiology, by way of review, we assume that the problems in functioning that we encompass in our conceptions of psychopathology are closely linked with under-developed, under-regulated, or under-integrated neural networks, and empirical studies documenting dysregulation in neural functioning across a range of disorders support these formulations. It follows that a fundamental task of psychotherapy is to generate experiential opportunities that restore and strengthen the integration of neural functions believed to underlie health, well-being, and adaptive functioning. In this sense, as I have observed, we can think of the core activities of psychotherapy as varieties of enriching experience that foster the growth of neurons and expand connections across neural networks, changing the structure and function of the brain.

Domains of Integration

Clinical scholars in the field of interpersonal neurobiology describe two fundamental domains of integration in their models of the networks believed to govern brain function, categorized according to vertical and horizontal axes. The vertical axis refers to the core structures of the brain: the brainstem, the limbic region, and the cerebral cortex. The horizontal axis refers to the right and left hemispheres of the brain. Researchers propose that the integration and coordination of neural networks linking these systems mediates our experience of sensation, emotion, imagery, cognition, behavior, and awareness, influencing states of self and capacities for emotional regulation, coping, health, and well-being.

Vertical Integration

The formative "drive toward integration" that Winnicott elaborates in his accounts of maturation bridges the core structures of the brain over the course of development, strengthening capacities to control reflexes and regulate emotion originating in the brainstem and limbic system. Top-down and bottom-up processing systems modulate our perceptions and reactions within the ranges of adaptive functioning; Eric Kandel likens them to the dial on the radio that controls the volume (2012).

In top-down forms of vertical integration, researchers propose, cortical functions process, organize, and regulate sensations, reflexes, impulses, and emotions arising in the brainstem and limbic system (Cozolino, 2017, p. 29). Top-down processing, carried out by inference and comparison to earlier experience preserved in memory, mediates perception, arousal, and states of self. Cognitive functions are instrumental in coping, guiding selection of "emotion focused" and "problem-focused" strategies (see Borden, 1991a, 1991b; Kandel, 2012; Lazarus & Folkman, 1984).

As we will see, therapists use a range of approaches believed to engage top-down mechanisms of integration, helping patients reappraise negative perceptions of experience in light of actual circumstances and realistic prospects, attempting to strengthen capacities to process information, reframe events, regulate emotion, and cope with challenges. The functions of the frontal cortex calm the amygdala and the sympathetic nervous system, reducing distress. Biological vulnerabilities, developmental delay, injury, or various forms of trauma may compromise the functioning of top-down systems, leading to difficulties in impulse control, emotional regulation, and focusing of attention.

Researchers have linked a range of bottom-up systems to structures in the cortex that influence perception, arousal, mood, attention, and learning; these systems, governed largely by genetic factors, release neurotransmitters that influence physiological and behavioral outcomes essential for the integrated functioning of the brain, health, and well-being. Although a full review of the core bottom-up systems is beyond the scope of this chapter, it is important to understand that they mediate a range of emotions and behaviors instrumental in subjective experience and relational life, including capacities for trust, bonding, empathy, happiness, sadness, and emotional regulation. As we will see, a variety of activities carry the potential to engage bottom-up systems, including breathing practices, meditation, walking, yoga, dance, and musical performance (for expanded accounts of bottom-up systems see Kandel, 2012; LeDoux, 2015; and Sapolsky, 2017).

Horizontal Integration

Although the corpus callosum links the left and right hemispheres of the brain, mediating our experience of perception, emotion, thought, language, and memory, they differ in fundamental respects; as noted, some researchers distinguish a "conscious left brain system" and an "unconscious right-brain system" proposing that the two hemispheres create "coherent, utterly different, and often incompatible versions of the world with competing priorities and values" (Schore, 2012, p. 8; see McGilchrist, 2009, for an expanded account of hemispheric laterality).

For more than a century, neurologists have assumed that language and verbal abilities are dependent on the left hemisphere. Pierre-Paul Broca and Carl Wernicke located critical language functions in the left region, and there is widespread agreement that this part of the brain is instrumental in conscious, verbal, rational, and serial modes of processing information. The left hemisphere categorizes perceptions based on inference and prior experience from a top-down process, as noted earlier, and it appears to be specialized for the regulation of well-established patterns of behavior in everyday life (Schore, 2019a, 2019b; Siegel, 2020).

The right hemisphere, on the other hand, is closely linked with unconscious, implicit, non-verbal, holistic, intuitive, and relational modes of information processing; it plays a major role in emotional arousal, having dense connections to the amygdala and the autonomic nervous system, mediating visceral reactions to experience. The functions of the right hemisphere underlie capacities to perceive holistic patterns, drawing on non-verbal realms of sensation, imagery, and sound. The right brain helps us get the gist of experiences and the fundamental meaning of events; as Siegel explains, rapidly associated images provide more immediate readings of experience, perceiving the world for "how it is" from a "bottom-up" perspective (Siegel, 2012, p. 256).

Accordingly, the specialization of the two hemispheres provides distinct modes of processing experience, and conceptions of horizontal integration help us consider the ways in which we engage differing capacities and functions across both regions of the brain in light of changing needs, tasks, and conditions. In order to relate the experience of my grandmother in the garden that I shared in the preceding chapter, for example, I must engage the conscious, linguistic functions of the left hemisphere and implicit memories and perceptual and emotional functions operating in the right hemisphere as I formulate the account. Horizontal integration is reflected in our ability to render experience into words and our capacity for real-time processing of sensations, emotions, images, and thoughts.

Schore has increasingly focused on the synchronized, right-lateralized forms of intersubjective communication and regulation of emotion in his reformulations of therapeutic action in the psychodynamic paradigm, expanding conceptions of projective identification, enactment, and regression in light of empirical findings in affective neuroscience and interpersonal neurobiology that document the crucial role of right hemisphere functions in change and growth. Following the developmental arrest of trauma, he proposes, the loosening of "top-down" left hemispheric control of the right hemisphere and engagement of deeper regions of the unconscious carry the potential to reinstate the maturation of the subjective self of the right brain, rebalancing the hemispheres (Schore, 2019b, p. 154).

Facilitating Neural Integration in Psychotherapy

Although the above models of brain function are highly schematized and simplified, failing to reflect the complexity of the synchronizations believed to link the regions of the connectome, they serve as heuristics in continuing efforts to explore basic mechanisms of change and growth in psychotherapy. In line with current understanding, researchers propose that therapists facilitate the integration of neural systems through the ongoing engagement of the language-based cognitive functions of the "top" cortical regions of the left hemisphere and the processing of unconscious, implicit, sensory and emotional realms of experience closely linked with the right hemisphere and the "bottom" regions of the brain (Cozolino, 2017; Kandel, 2018; Sapolsky, 2017; Schore, 2019a, 2019b; Siegel, 2010, 2020).

In focusing awareness on different aspects of our experience, researchers assume that we activate patterns of neural firing in regions of the brain associated with earlier events and current problems in functioning. The repeated processing of experience over the course of psychotherapy, linking the domains of sensation, emotion, imagery, thought, and behavior, is thought to generate new synaptic connections that lead to the reorganization of neural networks, strengthening the integration of core structures and functions throughout the brain in accordance with the principles of Hebbian learning and the dynamics of long-term potentiation (Cozolino 2017; Doidge, 2015; Kandel 2018; Siegel, 2020; Wallin 2007).

As we have seen, the subcortical regions of the brain—particularly the structures of the limbic system—are instrumental in regulating stress and emotion. Given our understanding of the evolution of the brain and the dynamics of neural functioning, in accord with the hierarchical model that John Hughlings Jackson proposed at the end of the 19th century, researchers assume that "bottom-up" processes, originating in the brain stem and other subcortical structures, exert a disproportionate influence over our experience of sensation, feeling, thought, and behavior (see LeDoux, 2015; Sapolsky, 2017; Wallin, 2007).

The cortical functions thought to be most influential in regulating the dynamics of inner experience and behavior are located in the middle prefrontal region, which is closely linked to the right hemisphere and the amygdala, modulating emotion and integrating information from the core structures of the brain. The other section of the cortex, the dorsolateral region, as noted earlier, is closely linked with the hippocampus and the linguistic functions of the left hemisphere, governing conscious processing and verbal formulations of experience.

In light of research findings documenting the influence of common factors on therapeutic outcomes reviewed in Chapter 1, it is reasonable to assume that all forms of psychotherapy carry the potential to engage the functions of both hemispheres and activate "top-down" and "bottom-up" systems of regulation through the core activities of help and care. As Rosenzweig emphasized in his seminal account of common factors believed to operate across divergent approaches, "there are inevitably certain unrecognized factors in any therapeutic situation" that may be "even more important than those being purposely employed" (1936, p. 412).

Even so, clinical scholars in the field of interpersonal neurobiology have proposed that certain approaches may be more or less likely to engage particular structures and functions of the brain instrumental in the processes that govern neural integration, emotional regulation, change, and growth. The techniques of free association developed in psychoanalytic psychotherapy and the experiential methods of processing somatic states and emotion that shape therapeutic action in the humanistic paradigm may engage the dynamics of implicit memory, bringing about change in sensation, feeling, and meaning, but fail to address patterns of thought and behavior that operate through the action of different networks. The techniques of cognitive-behavior therapy may alter explicit forms of thought and action but fail to reorganize the underlying neural networks that perpetuate vicious circles of feeling, thinking, and acting.

Some thinkers have proposed that classical cognitive approaches, emphasizing rational processing of experience, engage the dorsolateral region more fully than the middle prefrontal region, believed to play a fundamental role in the integration of neural structures and regulation of emotion. In light of the absence of networks bridging the dorsolateral region and the limbic system, David Wallin reasons, "top-down" approaches that focus only on thinking about feelings may fail to bring about long-term change. It is critical, he argues, to combine "top-down" methods and "bottom-up" approaches believed to engage the middle prefrontal region of the cortex, helping patients process and integrate somatic states, feelings, thoughts, and behavior in real time (2007, p. 81).

Wallin thinks of "interoceptive attention" as a form of mindfulness that helps patients ground themselves in the present, focusing on their immediate experience of sensation, feeling, thought, and behavior, strengthening capacities for emotional regulation. Jonathan Shedler speculates that traditional forms of cognitive-behavior therapy may be effective in part because skilled clinicians use a wider range of approaches and methods that have shaped practice in the psychodynamic tradition, focusing largely on emotion and the interactive experience of the therapeutic process (Shedler, 2010). Reviewing research in cognitive neuroscience, Drew Westen and Glenn Gabbard urge clinicians to consider a range of methods in their efforts to engage implicit and explicit domains of experience over the course of the therapeutic process, reasoning that the multiple systems of the brain, reflecting distinct anatomical structures, require different forms of intervention (Gabbard & Westen, 2003; Westen, 2005).

Researchers assume that all forms of therapy are effective to the degree that they enhance plasticity and neural integration, believing that the improvement and growth we see over the course of psychotherapy are closely linked to change in the structure and function of the brain (Cozolino, 2017; Schore, 2019a, 2019b; Siegel, 2020). As I noted in the introduction, recent reviews of research in the fields of neurogenetics, molecular biology, and brain imaging provide empirical support for the above proposals, documenting changes in gene expression, neurotransmitter metabolism, and enduring modifications in synaptic plasticity following therapeutic intervention (Glass, 2008; Kandel, 2012, 2018; Schore, 2019b; Siegel, 2020; Solms, 2018a, 2018b; for reviews see Borden, 2014).

Neuroplasticity, Therapeutic Action, and Change

Although William James, Sigmund Freud, and Santiago Ramon y Cajal introduced formulations of neuroplasticity in their accounts of the brain toward the end of the 19th century, modern neuroscientists came to believe that the core structures of the brain are "hardwired," fixed in accordance with the form and function of genetic codes, immutable by adulthood. Over the last two decades, however, researchers have rediscovered the ways in which the brain remains elastic and flexible, capable of change and growth across the course of life. Experience—patterns of activation—changes the brain.

The pioneering research of Eric Kandel, documenting the fundamental role of learning in gene expression and the development of neural structures in the marine snail *aplysia californica*, deepens our understanding of the dynamics of neuroplasticity and the ways in which the experiential opportunities of psychotherapy potentially expand and strengthen the networks that form the neural substrate of mind.

Kandel completed training in psychiatry and had planned to practice psychoanalysis before he decided to pursue a research career in neuroscience, and he began to explore the clinical implications of neuroplasticity decades before he received the Nobel Prize for his studies of the cellular mechanisms of learning and memory in 2000. Drawing on Cajal's theory that learning modifies the strength of synaptic connections between neurons, he proposed that different forms of learning generate different patterns of neural activity that change the strength of synaptic connections in particular ways. In 1979, in his account of "Psychotherapy and the single synapse," he explored the relevance of neuroplasticity for clinical practice, framing psychotherapy as a psychological and social influence that changes the brain. "It is only insofar as our words produce changes in each other's brains," Kandel proposed, "that psychotherapeutic intervention produces changes in patients' minds. From this perspective, the biological and psychological approaches are joined" (1979, p. 1037).

He had chosen the sea slug for his research because the neural memory structure of the snail is observable to the naked eye, allowing Kandel and his collaborators to map a series of networks and functions that they manipulated in classic conditioning experiments. In his studies of the snail, carried out over three decades, he found that the number of synapses doubles or triples as a result of learning.

Although the anatomical connections between neurons develop according to a definite plan, the strength and effectiveness of the connections are not fully determined by template genes. They can be altered by experience. In Kandel's account of neural development, experience activates the transcription of certain genes that facilitate the synthesis of proteins instrumental in the development of neural structures. Gene transcription mediates the ongoing growth of neurons, altering the structure and function of the cell. Experiential learning in the social surround continues to shape the development of the brain, modifying the molecular mechanisms that govern gene expression, determining when genes express themselves through the process of protein synthesis (Kandel, 1998, 2006, 2018). Nature and nurture, genetic action and experience, shape the development of the brain.

Kandel continued to explore the ways in which the experiential opportunities of psychotherapy potentially expand and strengthen the networks that form the neural substrate of mind. In an influential article, "A new intellectual framework for psychiatry," he proposed that the experiential learning that occurs over the course of psychotherapy carries the potential to bring about the comparable degrees of growth in neuronal and synaptic functioning that he had documented in his studies of the sea slug.

When psychotherapy brings about change and growth, he argued, "it presumably does so through learning, by producing changes in gene expression that alter the strength of synaptic connections, and structural changes that alter the anatomical patter of interconnections between nerve cells of the brain" (Kandel, 1998, p. 460). The interactive experience of psychotherapy, engaging the mental processes of mind, carries the potential to change the physical processes of the body.

The "regulation of gene expression by social factors makes all bodily functions, including all functions of the brain, susceptible to social influences," Kandel explains. "These social influences will be biologically incorporated in the altered expressions of specific genes in specific nerve cells in specific regions of the brain" (1998, p. 461).

> When a therapist speaks to a patient and the patient listens, the therapist is not only making eye contact and voice contact, but the action of neuronal machinery in the therapist's brain is having an indirect, and, one hopes, long-lasting effect on the neural machinery in the patient's brain and quite likely, vice versa. Insofar as our words produce changes in our patient's mind, it is likely that these psychotherapeutic interventions produce changes in the patient's brain. From this perspective, the biological and the sociopsychological approaches are joined.
>
> (1998, p. 466)

Kandel believes that psychological and social domains of understanding remain crucial as we continue to shape the science of mind, and he attributes causal factors to the dynamics of mental life and interactive experience in accord with the principles of non-reductive materialism, offering an integrative biopsychosocial perspective (see Kandel, 1999). The structure and function of the brain are shaped by experience unique to each individual, dependent on the person's particular experiential history (Milner, Squire & Kandel, 1998, p. 463).

Drawing on Kandel's research, clinical scholars in the field of interpersonal neurobiology have emphasized the recursive dynamics of the development of brain and mind across the life course (Howe & Lewis, 2005; Kandel, 2018). Our behavior shapes genetic expression and regulation, creating patterns of activation and neural connections that, in turn, influence how we feel, think, and act. As Siegel explains: "Experience, gene expression and gene regulation, mental activity, behavior, and continued interactions with the environment (experience) are tightly linked in a transactional set of processes" (2020, pp. 50–51). Genes and experience, nature and nurture, shape the development of the brain and mind. The structural changes may encompass the genesis of new neural tissue and expanded arborization of neurons, enhancing synaptic connectivity.

The transcription function of genes underlies our capacity for neuroplasticity across the course of life, and our conceptions of Hebbian learning and long-term potentiation provide heuristics for understanding the ways in which the core conditions of the therapeutic relationship and the experiential opportunities of help and care potentially promote the growth of neurons and expansion of neural networks, changing the structure and function of the brain.

Facilitating Processes and Experiential Learning in Psychotherapy

The above lines of study in the science of mind deepen our appreciation of the ways in which the experiential opportunities of psychotherapy potentially bring about change and growth across the foundational schools of thought. Drawing on developmental concepts and empirical findings in the fields of neuroscience and developmental psychology, psychotherapy research, and clinical observation, we can identify core elements of the therapeutic process that would appear to be fundamental in fostering neural plasticity, growth, and integration. I outline formulations in five areas that offer points of reference for our reviews of clinical theory and concepts of therapeutic action. In doing so I expand working hypotheses proposed by clinical scholars in the field of interpersonal neurobiology centering on four domains of experience believed to promote neuroplasticity: the core conditions of the therapeutic relationship; moderate levels of arousal or "optimal stress;" the activation of cognition and emotion; and the co-construction of narratives that foster an affirming sense of self and possibility (Cozolino, 2017; Schore, 2019b; Siegel, 2020). We will consider these ideas more fully in our discussions of theoretical concepts and case studies in the following chapters.

The Therapeutic Relationship, Interactive Experience, and the Constancy of Care in the Holding Environment

As we have seen, the attachment bond and early caretaking experience shape the architecture of the brain, playing a formative role in the development of core integrative and regulatory structures. In light of our growing appreciation of the dynamics of neuroplasticity, however, we assume that relational experience continues to mediate the organization and strength of neural connections throughout life. Converging lines of study in neuroscience suggest that the core conditions of the therapeutic relationship carry the potential to activate bonding processes instrumental in attachment, creating an optimal biochemical environment for neural plasticity (Cozolino, 2017; Schore, 2019b; Solms, 2018a).

In line with current research, clinical scholars propose that the empathic attunement and synchrony of the therapeutic relationship, the constancy of care in the holding environment, and the interactive experience of the therapeutic process—particularly forms of communication mediated by the right hemisphere —potentially reinstate neural growth and development, helping patients strengthen capacities to process and integrate subjective experience, regulate emotion, and negotiate the dynamics of relational life (Cozolino, 2017; Schore, 2019a, 2019b; Siegel, 2020).

Following developments in attachment research and affective neuroscience over the last decade, clinical scholars increasingly emphasize the role of unconscious, non-verbal, emotional processes rather than conscious, verbal, cognitive processes in their reformulations of therapeutic action, change and growth. What matters most, as Allan Schore has emphasized, is our *way of being* in the clinical situation, especially in times of vulnerability and fear.

The right hemisphere is critical in processing the "music" carried in our words, as Schore explains, urging clinicians to expand concepts of therapeutic action to encompass non-verbal domains of interactive experience that regulate bodily states and emotion. Prosody conveys nuances of meaning through variations in stress and pitch, independent of the grammar and words. The non-verbal elements of language—intonation, inflection, tone, pitch, force, and rhythm—evoke states of self, sometimes associated with implicit memories and reactions in early life. More broadly, non-verbal communication includes body movement, posture, gesture, and facial expression (see Dorpat, 2001, for an account of primary process communication). The right hemisphere mediates the more fundamental forms of communication in the therapeutic process, and right brain to right brain intersubjective transactions lie at the core of the therapeutic relationship, mediating what Louis Sander describes as "moments of meeting" between the clinician and the patient (Sander, 1992, cited in Schore, 2012, p. 39).

Challenge, Optimal Stress, and Emotion

Clinicians have recognized the crucial role of emotion in change and growth from the start of therapeutic practice. In their formulation of the cathartic method at the end of the 19th century, Freud and Josef Breuer proposed that "abreaction" of traumatic experiences in their full intensity would release "strangulated" emotion and alleviate symptoms that had perpetuated problems in functioning (see Chapter 4).

In developing his conceptual framework for psychotherapy, Jerome Frank proposed that emotional arousal facilitates change in a variety of ways (Frank & Frank, 1991, p. 46). The experience of emotion may strengthen the patient's motivation to engage in the therapeutic process; challenge patterns of defense; support efforts to process, formulate, and integrate experience, and facilitate the development of more functional ways of managing vulnerability and problems in living. In the domain of the humanities, Frank considers the potential importance of healing emotions generated by our experience of literature and art as well as creative arts therapies involving music, dance, painting, sculpting, and writing. We consider the therapeutic functions of these activities and practices further in Chapter 9.

As we will see, all therapeutic approaches intensify emotion through different methods and procedures. In psychodynamic psychotherapy, for example, clinicians challenge the dynamics of defense through exploration of emotion, processing of interactive experience, and interpretation of behavior. In classical cognitive approaches, clinicians challenge ways of processing and interpreting experience that fail to take account of actual circumstances and realistic prospects. Behavior therapists introduce methods of exposure in their efforts to help patients challenge avoidant behavior and engage feared domains of inner and outer experience that perpetuate problems in functioning.

Research findings indicate that moderate levels of arousal and "optimal stress" foster neurobiological conditions that promote plasticity, learning, and neural integration. Moderate levels of arousal activate the production of neurotransmitters and neural growth hormones believed to enhance long-term potentiation, learning, and cortical reorganization (for review of empirical findings see Cozolino, 2017). The ebb and flow of emotion over the course of therapy, as Cozolino observes, "reflects the underlying rhythms of growth and change" (2017, p. 48). Acceptance, support, and challenge are thought to be crucial elements in change and growth across all forms of psychotherapy.

Engagement of Sensation, Emotion, Imagery, Cognition, and Behavior in the Therapeutic Process

Clinical scholars have proposed that simultaneous or alternating engagement of emotion and cognition fosters the development and reorganization of under-integrated neural networks believed to perpetuate dysregulation, dissociation, and dysfunction; I expand this formulation to encompass the domains of sensation, imagery, and behavior in order to take account of the wider range of phenomena in human experience. As we repeatedly focus our attention on various aspects of experience, researchers assume that we activate neural firing associated with conditions and circumstances, creating new synaptic connections, reorganizing neural networks. Presumably, the engagement of under-developed or under-regulated networks fosters the integration of neural structures and functions in accord with Hebb's proposal that activation of neural circuits in real time creates or strengthens connections that link and coordinate their functioning (see Cozolino, 2017, p. 49). As we will see, Freud prefigured these findings in elaborating his concepts of therapeutic action, described most fully in his seminal paper "Remembering, repeating, and working through" (1914/1958; see further discussion in Chapter 4).

The capacity to tolerate emotion and regulate states of self creates conditions for neural growth and integration across the course of life; as Cozolino observes, we can think of emotional regulation as a crucial outcome of help and care across all therapeutic approaches because it allows us to make use of experiential opportunities and relationships that foster growth (2017). The greater the integration of neural networks, presumably, the greater the capacity to experience, tolerate, and make use of sensations, feelings, images, and thoughts previously dissociated or managed through other defensive processes.

Formulations of Experience and Co-Construction of Narratives

Language is a core constituent of neural and psychological development, instrumental in the formation of memory and self-identity, and we can think of narratives as natural cognitive and linguistic forms that facilitate ongoing efforts to formulate experience and create meaning across the course of life (Borden, 1992, 2000, 2010; Bruner, 1990). Although we remain largely unaware of the interpretive processes that underlie the construction of life stories, ongoing narratives about self and life events serve as filters for perception, processing, organization, and understanding of experience. From a developmental perspective, personal narratives help us preserve a sense of coherence, continuity, and unity in sense of self and identity through the life course, helping us define who we have been, who we are, and who we may become in the future.

Researchers propose that ongoing formulations of experience and co-creation of narrative accounts over the course of the therapeutic process engages the functions of the left and right hemispheres, fostering the integration of neural networks throughout the brain. As Siegel explains, the autonoetic, analogical, context-dependent, mentalizing functions of the right hemisphere shape the themes and imagery of the narrative process, while the left hemisphere mediates interpretive and linguistic processing of content. He proposes:

> The left hemisphere's drive to understand cause-effect relationships is a primary motivation of the narrative process. Coherent narratives, however, require participation of both the interpreting left hemisphere and the mentalizing right hemisphere. Coherent narratives are created through interhemispheric integration.
>
> (2020, p. 455)

Enriching Relationships, Activities, Practices, and Places in the Outer World

Beyond the experiential opportunities of the therapeutic process itself, we increasingly recognize the crucial role of enriching relationships, activities, and practices in everyday life that potentially foster neural integration, change, growth, and well-being. Clinicians describe a range of "bottom-up" practices believed to engage subcortical regions of sensation and emotion, including meditation, walking, yoga, tai chi, prayer, and artistic and musical activities (Van der Kolk, 2014; Wallin, 2007; Walsh, 2011).

Researchers continue to explore the experience of place and nature as a potential source of healing, change, and growth. The emerging field of environmental neuroscience is documenting the ways in which the features of natural surrounds influence neural function, mood, well-being, and patterns of behavior (for review of orienting perspectives and empirical findings see Berman, Stier & Akcelik, 2019; for reviews of research on the healing functions of place, see Sternberg, 2009; for review of research on the effects of nature on cognition and mood, see Williams, 2017). I explore these concerns further in discussion of integrative approaches in Chapter 9.

Neuroscience, the Person, and Clinical Pragmatism

Converging lines of study in the science of mind continue to strengthen empirical support for the core processes of psychotherapy, validating the importance of ideas and methods across the foundational schools of thought. Growing understanding of the dynamics of attachment, implicit and explicit memory, and the mechanisms of neuroplasticity across the life course promises to strengthen the conceptual and empirical foundations of therapeutic practices.

The fields of neuroscience deepen our understanding of the connections between the brain and our changing experience of sensation, emotion, thought, and behavior, just as they strengthen our appreciation of the range of conditions that perpetuate vulnerability and problems in living. Conceptual syntheses and empirical findings offer heuristics that strengthen our formulations of what is the matter and what carries the potential to help, challenging clinicians to consider a wide range of approaches. Developments in the science of mind enrich our thinking about the ways in which various forms of therapeutic action potentially bring about change and growth, offering points of reference across the schools of thought as we consider core elements and different ways of working over the course of psychotherapy.

In more reductive renderings of help and care, some clinicians have proposed that we will come to think of psychotherapy as a biological science or "applied neuroscience" that "rewires" the brain (Cozolino, 2017). Some researchers predict that, in time, we will be able to select specific techniques of intervention and monitor the progress of psychotherapy through the methods of neuroimaging (Kandel, 2018). Such sweeping proposals are problematic in light of the pragmatic values and concerns outlined earlier. However promising scholars and psychotherapists find recent developments in the science of mind, it is crucial to challenge a "technical rationality" and avoid reductive or formulaic applications of research findings that would violate the principles and values of clinical pragmatism, realizing the complexities, ambiguities, and contingencies of therapeutic practice.

As psychotherapists our fundamental concern is not the neuron but the individual, the "human person"—"the most interesting entity known to exist in the universe," as the novelist Marilynne Robinson reminds us in her critiques of neuroscience (2012, p. 144). We cannot expect neurobiology alone to explain the course or outcome of the therapeutic process. In accord with the principles of clinical pragmatism, we must consider a range of paradigms and a multitude of concepts as we work to understand people, problems in living, and what carries the potential to help, taking account of differences in personality and temperament, the nature of subjective experience, capacities and skills, experiential learning, and the irreducible features of the therapeutic process that defy classification or categorization. As converging lines of study in the science of mind and psychotherapy show, it is the *experience* of help and care—the ways in which we make use of different elements over the course of the therapeutic process—that carries the potential for healing, change, and growth. "An ounce of experience," Dewey reminds us, "is better than a ton of theory simply because it is only in experience that any theory has vital and verifiable significance" (1916, p. 144).

References

Berman, M. G., Stier, A. J. & Akcelik, G. N. (2019). Environmental neuroscience. *American Psychologist*, 1 (3), 1039–1052.

Borden, W. (1991a). Beneficial outcomes in adjustment following HIV seropositivity. *Social Service Review*, 65 (3), 434–449.

Borden, W. (1991b). Stress, appraisal, and coping in spouses of demented elderly: Predictors of psychological well-being. *Social Work Research and Abstracts*, 27 (1), 14–21.

Borden, W. (1992). Narrative perspectives in psychosocial intervention following adverse life events. *Social Work*, 37 (2), 135–141.

Borden, W. (2000). *The life review in context: Theory, research, and practice. Issues in Aging*. Chicago, IL: Center for Applied Gerontology.

Borden, W. (2010). Taking multiplicity seriously: Pluralism, pragmatism, and integrative perspectives in social work practice, in W. Borden (Ed.), *Reshaping theory in contemporary social work* (pp. 3–28). New York: Columbia University Press.

Borden, W. (2014). Neuroscience, therapeutic action, and clinical pragmatism. Rhoda Sarnat Lecture, Oct. 24, University of Chicago, Chicago, IL.

Bruner, J. (1990). *Acts of meaning*. Cambridge, MA: Harvard University Press.

Cozolino, L. (2017). *The neuroscience of psychotherapy*, 3rd edn. New York: Norton.

Dewey, J. (1916). *Democracy and education: An introduction to the philosophy of education*. New York: Macmillan.

Doidge, N. (2015). *The brain's way of healing: Remarkable discoveries and recoveries from the frontiers of neuroplasticity*. New York: Viking.

Dorpat, T. L. (2001). Primary process communication. *Psychoanalytic Inquiry*, 3, 448–463.

Frank, J. & Frank J. (1991). *Healing and persuasion*. Baltimore, MD: John Hopkins University Press.

Freud, S. (1914/1958). Remembering, repeating, and working through, in *Further recommendations in the techniques of psychoanalysis II*, in J. Strachey (Ed. and Trans.), *The standard edition of the compete psychological works of Sigmund Freud*, Vol. 12 (pp. 145–156). London: Hogarth Press.

Gabbard, G. & Westen, D. (2003). Rethinking therapeutic action. *International Journal of Psychoanalysis*, 84, 235–250.

Glass, R. M. (2008). Psychodynamic psychotherapy and research evidence: Bambi survives Godzilla? *Journal of the American Medical Association*, 300 (13), 1587–1589.

Howe, M. L. & Lewis, M. (2005). The importance of dynamic systems approaches for understanding development. *Developmental Review*, 25 (3–4), 247–251.

Kandel, E. (1979). Psychotherapy and the single synapse: The impact of psychiatric thought on neurobiological research. *New England Journal of Medicine*, 301 (19), 1028–1037.

Kandel, E. (1998). A new intellectual framework for psychiatry. *American Journal of Psychiatry*, 155 (4), 457–469.

Kandel, E. (1999). Biology and the future of psychoanalysis: A new intellectual framework for psychiatry revisited. *American Journal of Psychiatry*, 156 (4), 505–524.

Kandel, E. (2006). *In search of memory: The emergence of a new science of mind*. New York: Norton.

Kandel, E. (2012). *The age of insight*. New York: Random House.

Kandel, E. (2018). *The disordered mind*. New York: Farrar, Straus & Giroux.

Lazarus, R. & Folkman, S. (1984). *Stress, appraisal, and coping*. New York: Springer.

LeDoux, J. (2015). *Anxious*. New York: Viking.

McGilchrist, I. (2009). *The master and his emissary: The divided brain and the making of the western world*. New Haven, CT: Yale University Press.

Milner, B., Squire, L. & Kandel, E. (1998). Cognitive neuroscience and the study of memory. *Neuron*, 3, 445–468.

Pribram, K. H. (1991). *Brain and perception: Holonomy and structure in figural processing*. Hillsdale, NJ: Erlbaum.

Robinson, M. (2012). *When I was a child I read books*. New York: Farrar, Straus & Giroux.

Rosenzweig, S. (1936). Some implicit common factors in diverse methods of psychotherapy. *American Journal of Orthopsychiatry*, 6 (3), 412–415.

Sander, L. (1992). Letter to the editor. *International Journal of Psychoanalysis*, 73, 582–584.

Sapolsky, R. (2017). *Behave*. New York: Penguin.

Schore, A. (2012). *The science of the art of psychotherapy*. New York: Norton.

Schore, A. (2019a). *The development of the unconscious mind*. New York: Norton.

Schore, A. (2019b). *Right brain psychotherapy*. New York: Norton.

Shedler, J. (2010). The efficacy of psychodynamic psychotherapy. *American Psychologist*, 65 (2), 98–109.

Siegel, D. (2010). *The mindful therapist: A clinician's guide to mindsight and neural integration*. New York: Norton.

Siegel, D. (2012). *The developing mind*, 2nd edn. New York: Guilford.

Siegel, D. (2020). The developing mind, 3rd edn.New York: Guilford.

Solms, M. (2018a). The scientific standing of psychoanalysis. *British Journal of Psychiatry International*, 15, 5–8.

Solms, M. (2018b). The neurobiological underpinnings of psychoanalytic theory and therapy. *Frontiers in Behavioral Neuroscience*, 12, 294.

Sternberg, E. (2009). *Healing spaces: The science of place and well-being*. Cambridge, MA: Harvard University Press.

Van der Kolk, B. (2014). *The body keeps the score: Brain, mind, and body in the healing of trauma*. New York: Penguin.

Wallin, D. (2007). *Attachment in psychotherapy*. New York: Guilford.

Walsh, R. (2011). Lifestyle and mental health. *American Psychologist*, 6 (7), 579–592.

Westen, D. (2005). Implications of research in cognitive neuroscience for psychodynamic psychotherapy, in G. Gabbard, J. Beck & J. Holmes (Eds.), *Oxford textbook of psychotherapy* (pp. 43–48). New York: Oxford University Press.

Williams, F. (2017). *The nature fix*. New York: Norton.

Winnicott, D. W. (1960/1965). The theory of the parent-infant relationship, in D. W. Winnicott, *The maturational process and the facilitating environment* (pp. 37–55). New York: International Universities Press.

Winnicott, D. W. (1963/1965). A theory of psychiatric disorder. *The maturational process and the facilitating environment* (pp. 230–242). New York: International Universities Press.

Part III
Clinical Theories and Therapeutic Action

> Everything factual is already theory....The blueness of the sky reveals the basic law of chromatics. Don't go looking for anything beyond phenomena: they are themselves what they teach.
>
> –Goethe

Over the last three decades clinical scholars have come to appreciate the strengths and limitations of different approaches developed within the foundational schools of thought, exploring shared concerns and points of emphasis, and practitioners continue to combine ideas and methods from a range of perspectives in their efforts to expand concepts of therapeutic action and strengthen the outcomes of help and care. Thinkers have drawn on psychodynamic, behavioral, cognitive, and humanistic paradigms in fashioning integrative models of practice.

By way of example, Marsha Linehan joined behavioral and cognitive approaches with relational concepts and Buddhist mindfulness practices in developing her influential model of dialectical behavior therapy (Linehan, 1993). William Miller bridged the person-centered perspective of Carl Rogers and cognitive-behavioral methods in shaping his conceptions of motivational interviewing (Miller & Rollnick, 2012). Paul Wachtel continues to develop a pragmatic approach that links core concepts in relational psychoanalysis with behavioral, cognitive, experiential, and systemic perspectives, extending earlier integrations of psychoanalytic ideas and behavioral therapy (Wachtel, 2014).

I strongly support efforts to deepen our understanding of core processes believed to operate across the major schools of thought and to combine concepts and methods in practical, flexible approaches to help and care. In following the principles of clinical pragmatism, as we have seen, we consider the contributions of our "purist" thinkers and models of practice selectively in light of the particular needs of the clinical situation, joining ideas and methods from divergent perspectives that would be considered incompatible in more idealized renderings of the therapeutic endeavor.

In accord with the pluralist orientation of clinical pragmatism, however, it is crucial to preserve the distinct identities of the foundational schools of thought and to develop an appreciation of the concerns and values that influence different ways of seeing, understanding, and acting. A range of intellectual traditions and philosophical perspectives have shaped our paradigms of therapeutic action. Our classical behavioral approaches originate in positivist conceptions of science, for example, while humanistic perspectives are closely linked with phenomenology. Although the earliest versions of cognitive therapy emphasized notions of rationality and objective truth, contemporary models of practice draw largely on constructivism, postmodern thought, and the science of mind. In light of fundamental philosophical differences our theories of psychotherapy are incommensurable, operating as distinct systems of thought that cannot be integrated.

The foundational schools of psychotherapy set forth compelling accounts of the human situation, focusing our attention on overlapping realms of experience from different points of view, introducing a variety of root meta-phors, values, concerns, purposes, models, and methods that influence what we say and do in the clinical situation. If each paradigm fails to capture the varieties and complexities of our experience, all are crucial because they pro-pose different ways of attending, understanding, and acting, helping us appreciate the implications of divergent ideas by pressing them to their limits.

Without a solid grounding in the theories of psychotherapy, I argued in the introduction, we risk the dogmatic embrace of a single paradigm, a willy-nilly eclecticism, or reductive, mechanized approaches to treatment by protocol, lacking conceptual foundations for critical thinking as we negotiate the com-plexities and ambiguities of the clinical situation, failing to understand the ele-ments we are trying to integrate and why.

In the third part of the book we explore orienting perspectives and concepts of therapeutic action that shape understanding and practice in the psychody-namic, behavioral, cognitive, and humanistic schools of thought. In doing so, we trace the evolution of therapeutic practice in each paradigm and consider the ways in which recent developments in the science of mind have deepened our understanding of core processes believed to facilitate change and growth in accord with the principles and values of clinical pragmatism. As we approach our therapeutic practice from a pragmatic point of view, we come to appreciate the distinctive features of different orientations, shared concerns, and basic principles of help and care that often remain obscured by ideological differ-ences, parochialism, and factionalism among the different schools of thought.

Given the influence of psychoanalysis in the development of theory and practice across the paradigms of psychotherapy, I begin Part III with an account of the psychodynamic tradition. In Chapter 4 I focus on the depth psychologies of Sigmund Freud and C. G. Jung. In Chapter 5 I trace the emergence of relational perspectives in contemporary psychoanalysis. I con-tinue with reviews of the behavioral, cognitive, and humanistic traditions in Chapters 6–8. In Chapter 9 I present two cases and consider the ways in which orienting perspectives in the foundational schools of thought, neuroscience, and clinical pragmatism strengthen our understanding of essential concerns in therapeutic action.

References

Goethe, J. W. (1829/1998). *Maxims and reflections*, P. Hutchinson (Ed.), Elisabeth Stopp (Trans.). London: Penguin.

Linehan, M. (1993). *Cognitive treatment of borderline personality disorder*. New York: Guilford.

Miller, W. & Rollnick, S. (2012). *Motivational interviewing: Helping people change*, 3rd edn. New York: Guilford.

Wachtel, P. (2014). *Cyclical psychodynamics and the contextual self*. New York: Routledge.

4 The Psychodynamic Paradigm

Depth Psychology

> Natural science combines two worlds, the physical and the psychic. Psychology does this only in so far as it is psychophysiology.
>
> –C. G. Jung

Critiques of psychoanalysis and reformulations of psychodynamic thought have brought about major shifts in theoretical perspectives, empirical research, and therapeutic practice over the last three decades. The growing emphasis on interdisciplinary study, bridging work in science and the humanities, continues to enlarge the scope of understanding. Emerging perspectives have been shaped by empirical findings in the fields of genetics, evolutionary biology, neuroscience, cognitive psychology, experimental psychology, developmental psychology, personality psychology, social psychology, and cultural anthropology. Some scholars think of psychoanalysis as a science of mind; others view it as an interpretive or hermeneutic discipline. Thinkers have increasingly centered on conceptions of self, relationship, and social life in their reformulations of theory, emphasizing the multiplicity and complexity of human experience. Research findings across the fields of neuroscience and developmental psychology provide strong support for the core propositions of psychodynamic understanding, emphasizing the crucial role of attachment and relational life in the development of the self and the dynamics of unconscious emotional and cognitive processes (Fonagy, Gergely, Jurist & Target, 2018; Glass, 2008; Kandel, 2018; Luborsky & Barrett, 2006; Schore, 2019a, 2019b; Solms, 2018a, 2018b; Westen, 1998, 2005).

Clinical scholars have identified core processes and techniques that distinguish psychodynamic psychotherapy from other forms of therapy explored in the following chapters. Matthew Blagys and Mark Hilsenroth carried out an analysis of empirical studies in the PsychLit database, reviewing session recordings and transcripts, and described the defining features of psychodynamic therapy as follows: 1) focus on emotion and expression of feelings; 2) exploration of attempts to avoid distressing feelings and thoughts; 3) identification of recurring themes and patterns in feelings, thoughts, actions, and relationships; 4) exploration of past experiences in light of current concerns and problems in living; 5) focus on interpersonal experiences; 6) emphasis on the therapeutic relationship and the dynamics of interactive experience; and 7) exploration of subjective experience (Blagys & Hilsenroth, 2000). A group of experienced clinicians corroborated these findings in constructing a prototype of the ideal version of psychodynamic psychotherapy (Shedler, 2010; Solms, 2018b).

In the domain of clinical research, outcome studies continue to document the efficacy and effectiveness of psychodynamic psychotherapy. In an influential review of meta-analyses representing the most rigorous evaluations of psychodynamically oriented therapy, Jonathan Shedler reported that the effect sizes are as large as those found for other forms of intervention widely regarded as "empirically supported" and "evidence-based" (2010, p. 98). As he details in his account, randomized controlled trials support the efficacy of psychodynamic therapy for a range of conditions, including depression, personality disorders, post-traumatic stress disorder, anxiety and panic disorders, eating disorders, and substance-related disorders (see Blatt, Zuroff & Hawley, 2009; Fonagy, Roth & Higgitt, 2005; Gibbons, Crits-Christoph & Hearon, 2008; Leichsenring, 2009; Leichsenring & Rabung, 2009; Westen, Novotny & Thompson-Brenner, 2004). Further, follow-up studies indicate that patients who receive psychodynamic therapy not only maintain gains over time but continue to improve after treatment ends, whereas the benefits of other forms of therapy tend to decay over time. Recent meta-analyses provide additional support for these findings, showing consistent trends toward larger effect sizes at follow-up, suggesting that psychodynamic approaches engage core processes that continue to foster change and growth after the end of therapy (Solms, 2018b). Clinicians continue to integrate ideas and methods from other paradigms of psychotherapy in their efforts to broaden the scope of practice, engage a more diverse range of patients, strengthen the empirical foundations of therapeutic action, and improve the outcomes of help and care.

Even so, we find surprisingly little consideration of psychodynamic theory, research, or practice methods in advanced training programs across the fields of psychiatry, psychology, social work, and counseling. Many researchers, educators, and practitioners continue to reject psychodynamic perspectives in view of perceived conflicts with scientific conceptions of psychotherapy and the growing emphasis on technical procedures in evidence-based practice. Some clinical scholars have little knowledge of recent developments in psychodynamic theory and research, and their critiques of the psychoanalytic paradigm fail to reflect the range of empirical findings, relational approaches, social and cultural perspectives, and pragmatic concerns that have shaped contemporary understanding and practice. Widespread ignorance and neglect of research findings corroborating the basic propositions of psychodynamic theory, and the evidence generated by process and outcome research on psychodynamic psychotherapy continues to perpetuate these unfortunate gaps in understanding (Borden, 2009; Borden & Clark, 2012; Shedler, 2006, 2010, 2015; Solms, 2018a, 2018b; Weinberg & Westen, 2001; Westen, 1998, 2005; Westen & Gabbard, 2002a, 2002b).

Toward the end of the 20th century clinical scholars had come to distinguish two fundamental perspectives in their accounts of psychodynamic thought: the drive paradigm, based on Sigmund Freud's classical instinct theory, and the relational paradigm, which centers on the fundamental role of attachment, relationship, and social life in human experience (Greenberg & Mitchell, 1983). Although relational perspectives have shaped contemporary understanding and practice, the first generation of psychoanalytic thinkers continues to provide crucial points of reference across the broader psychodynamic tradition. As a starting point, accordingly, I explore the depth psychology of Freud and C. G. Jung, outlining the development of their thought and concepts of therapeutic action. I show how they prefigure recent developments in the science of mind and introduce pragmatic principles of clinical practice. I review the emergence of the relational paradigm and concepts of therapeutic action that shape contemporary understanding and practice in Chapter 5.

Freud and Psychoanalysis

Freud founded a discipline, introduced successive models of the mind, and created new methods of psychotherapy. If we find the fundamental propositions of his drive psychology deeply problematic, other formulations have become so much a part of everyday life that we fail to recognize their origins in his writings—implicit, unarticulated assumptions about ourselves and our habits of mind. Practitioners rediscover the phenomenal accuracy and clinical value of his observations, coming to see the ways in which his early accounts of trauma, the dynamics of the unconscious, the workings of memory, and essential concerns in the clinical situation prefigure understanding and practice in our time.

Eric Kandel, Allan Schore, Mark Solms, and other scholars in the science of mind have characterized their research as a continuation of Freud's attempts to establish an empirical psychology at the end of the 19th century, showing how the *Project for a scientific psychology*, his early effort to create a neural model of the mind, anticipates fundamental developments in the fields of modern neuroscience. His account, illustrated by his sketches of neural networks thought to govern unconscious processes, explores the domains of perception, consciousness, attention, cognition, wishes, dreams, sexuality, and defense, seeking to formulate an understanding of the dynamics of the brain and mind. A decade before Charles Sherrington had given synapses their name, Freud proposed that points of communication between nerve cells, "contact barriers," could be altered by learning, prefiguring conceptions of neuroplasticity. Karl Pribram and Merton Gill, writing in the 1970s, predicted that researchers working to bridge the neurological and the psychological would come to think of the *Project* as a "Rosetta Stone" (1976).

While historical accounts of Freud's contributions make sharp distinctions between his work as a neuroanatomist, neurologist, and psychoanalyst, the culture that shaped his early scientific training in medical school continued to influence his thinking and practice over the course of his career, and he remained steadfast in his belief that mental life is governed by the complex functioning of the brain. He was deeply moved by his readings of Charles Darwin and Goethe's *Ode to nature*, he tells us in his *Autobiographical study*, deciding to abandon his plan to study law and pursue training in medicine (1925/1989).

As a neuroanatomist working in the physiology laboratory of Ernst von Brucke at the University of Vienna, he embraced the vision of a positivist science advanced by his mentor and his contemporaries, Hermann von Helmholtz, Emil du Bois, and Carl Ludwig. They rejected notions of vitalism and the life force set forth in the romantic philosophy of nature that had shaped the teaching of physiology in medical education at the time and embraced the physical sciences, seeking to create a reductionist, analytic version of biology. Freud came to believe that all psychological phenomena originate in neurophysiological processes, assuming a mechanical relation between brain and mind, proposing that we can think of the person as a dynamic system governed by the laws of nature. He set out to establish "a psychology which shall be called a natural science: that is, to represent psychical processes as quantitatively determinate states of specifiable material particles..." (1895/1966, p. 295).

Two experiences were formative in shaping Freud's emerging conceptions of mind and therapeutic practice: his collaboration with Josef Breuer, a colleague in Brucke's laboratory, and his study with Jean-Martin Charcot, one of the leading neurologists in Europe, who had developed diagnostic procedures and therapeutic methods to treat the symptoms of neurosis at the Saltpetriere hospital in Paris.

Over the course of his research at Brucke's Institute of Physiology, Freud came to know Breuer, a cultured Viennese physician who embraced the analytic biology of Brucke and his contemporaries. Breuer had treated a patient known as Anna O.—later identified as Bertha Pappenheim, a feminist and one of the founders of the social work movement in Germany—during Freud's last two years at the Institute, between 1880 and 1882.

Breuer related that the adolescent had developed classic symptoms of hysteria while caring for her father. She reported the loss of sensation and motor paralysis of the left side of her body, difficulties in speech and hearing, and loss of consciousness. He placed her under hypnosis, following procedures that Charcot had developed to treat the symptoms of hysteria. Although the hypnotic procedure itself proved unsuccessful, Pappenheim found herself talking about her symptoms while in the altered state. Following her lead, Breuer encouraged her to continue processing her experience and found that her symptoms receded as she related the circumstances of their origin. She recounted how her father had rested his head on her left side, now paralyzed, as he was dying of a tubercular abscess in his lungs.

"It turned out that all her symptoms," Freud later recalled in his *Autobiographical study*, "went back to moving events which she had experienced while nursing her father; that is to say, her symptoms had a meaning and they were residues or reminiscences of those emotional situations… When the patient recalled a situation of this kind… with a free expression of emotion, the mental act which she had originally suppressed, the symptom was abolished and did not return" (Freud, 1925/1989, p. 12). The origins of her symptoms lay in the traumatic events of her past, as Freud explained in his account of the treatment. Anna O. called this "chimney sweeping," her "talking cure"; Breuer called it "catharsis."

Breuer's account of Anna O. deepened Freud's interest in the treatment of mental conditions, and he made arrangements to study with Charcot at the Saltpetriere in Paris in autumn of 1885 and spring of 1886. He worked in his laboratory and attended his clinical demonstrations, where he used hypnotic suggestion to induce and alleviate traumatic paralyses. When he returned to Vienna in 1887 he asked Breuer to teach him the methods he had developed in his treatment of Anna O.

In his attempts to clarify the etiology and mechanisms of the range of problems in functioning he encountered in his practice as a neurologist, Freud found that organic symptoms followed patterns that corresponded to neuroanatomy, consistent with the established understanding of the distribution of nerves, tracts, and regions of the brain. Symptoms originating in mental conditions, however, operated independently of the nervous system, as if anatomy did not exist. He came to appreciate the ways in which unconscious mental processes could influence behavior over the course of his fellowship. He realized the crucial role of psychological understanding in efforts to provide help and care: "The signs of (neurotic) illness originate from nothing other than a change in the action of their minds upon their bodies and the immediate cause of their disorders is to be looked for in their minds" (Freud, 1890, p. 286).

Freud encouraged Breuer to prepare an account of his treatment of Anna O., reconstructed from memory almost 14 years later, and it became the prototype of the cathartic method. In their pioneering work, *Studies in hysteria*, published in 1895, Breuer and Freud traced the origins of a range of problems in functioning to traumatic experience. They proposed that memories of traumatic events are dissociated from conscious experience, and the emotion associated with the experience is converted to somatic symptoms. What is left in awareness, they theorized, is a symbol that is connected with traumatic events through unconscious associative networks. If the patient can bring implicit memories of traumatic experience to awareness and process the "strangulated" emotion associated with events, the affect is "discharged" and symptoms recede. The goal of treatment, in Freud's earliest formulation of psychotherapy, was to alleviate symptoms through the processing and integration of traumatic experience; he called the expression of the repressed emotion associated with the symptoms "abreaction" (Breuer & Freud, 1893–1895/1955).

Freud drew on Darwin and evolutionary biology as he continued to develop his conceptions of mind, shifting the focus of his theorizing from trauma to the dynamics of instinctual life and unconscious forces, coming to create what Frank Sulloway has called a "genetic psychobiology" (1979). He proposed instinctual drive as the core constituent of psychic life, believing that the most fundamental human motives are rooted in biology. In his model of the mind the origins of pathogenic experience lie not in repressed memories of traumatic events, but most deeply in the vicissitudes of instinctual life; maladaptive ways of negotiating intrapsychic conflict precipitate problems in living. In fashioning his drive psychology, Freud came to privilege instinct over relational and social life, fantasy processes over perception of actual events, and psychic reality over actual experience in the outer world, thereby establishing the defining features of classical psychoanalysis (Borden, 2009; for an expanded discussion see Mitchell, 1988, pp. 41–62).

In his topographic model of the mind, introduced in *The interpretation of dreams* at the turn of the century, Freud outlined three domains of mental life: the unconscious, encompassing motivations, feelings, and thoughts that originate in the dynamics of instinctual life; the preconscious, the region of feelings and thoughts that are accessible to awareness through the focusing of attention; and the conscious realm of perceptions, feelings, and thoughts that are in awareness at the moment. He described two forms of psychic functioning: primary process, operating out of awareness, mediating the realms of dreams and fantasy, and secondary process, operating in the domain of consciousness, governing the executive functions of the ego and the dynamics of rational, reflective thinking (Freud, 1900/1953).

In his revised theory of mind, Freud introduced two ideas that would shape the course of psychoanalytic understanding. First, he had come to believe that emotional and cognitive processes operate largely out of awareness, and he proposed that most of our mental life is unconscious, viewing conscious feelings and thoughts as the exception rather than the rule. Second, he argued that mental events do not occur by chance but follow the principle of psychic determinism. In accordance with our current understanding of brain function, he assumed that associations in memory are causally linked; presumably, associative connections govern unconscious and conscious domains of experience through different neural structures. However irrational neurotic symptoms may seem, he proposed, they have meaning and *make sense* in light of the concrete particulars of earlier experience and the dynamics of psychic life.

Freud continued to revise his formulations of the mind over the next two decades, introducing the structural model in *The ego and the id* (1923/1961). He described three core structures of personality: the id, the ego, and the superego. He moved beyond the criterion of consciousness that had shaped his earlier version of the topographic model and categorized mental processes on the basis of their functions and purposes, centering on conflict between fulfillment of instinctual needs, the dictates of conscience, and the demands of reality. The id (the "it," in the original German, a term Freud drew from Nietzsche) represents the biological substrates of psychological experience. Freud thought of this region as the source of raw, unstructured instinctual forces that press for expression; it operates unconsciously, governed by the pleasure principle. In his earliest formulations of drive psychology Freud centered on the sexual instinct; in a revision of his theory in 1920, having witnessed the brutality of World War I, he proposed an aggressive instinct as well. The ego or "I," the conscious sense of self, is instrumental in perception, governing executive functions in accordance with the reality principle. As such it mediates the dynamics of instinctual experience, conscience, and the realities of the social surround. In the domain of neuroscience, we find points of connection with current formulations of the executive functions of the prefrontal cortex, as described in Chapter 2. He thought of the superego as the moral agency, formed through identifications with the values of parents and social attitudes, mediating conflict between the id and the ego. The three structures of personality regulate the dynamics of emotion, thought, and behavior in adaptive functioning (see Kandel, 2012, for expanded accounts).

Therapeutic Action

Although Freud introduced successive models of the mind in his efforts to create a unified theory of personality, psychopathology, and therapeutic action, he worked as a clinician from the mid-1880s onward, focused on the concrete particularities of people and problems in functioning, and he outlines what we have come to think of as basic principles and pragmatic considerations in all forms of psychotherapy. He emphasizes the crucial functions of the therapeutic alliance; a shared understanding of what is the matter and the focus of treatment; active provisions of support and education; recognition and management of transference reactions; and exploration of defensive behaviors, which often take the form of resistance (Breuer & Freud, 1893–1895/1955; see Borden, 1999, 2000, 2009; and Brendel, 2006, for accounts of Freud's clinical pragmatism).

In his earliest formulations of neurosis, as described earlier, he assumed that symptoms originate in repressed memories of traumatic experience. The goal of therapy was to help the patient recover memories, process emotions associated with the events, and integrate the experience into the present sense of self and life story. As he revised his theory of mind, however, he broadened the scope of the therapeutic endeavor, shifting the focus of his concern from the treatment of symptoms to the reorganization of personality itself. In refashioning his formulations of neurosis he focused on conceptions of impulse, anxiety, defense, and conflict.

He came to think of neurosis as a closed system of drives and defenses, working to understand the ways in which underlying conflict precipitates symptoms, constricts ways of being and relating, and perpetuates problems in living. The fundamental task of psychoanalysis, he proposed, is to help patients explore unconscious conflicts that perpetuate problems in living and to develop more functional ways of mediating inner experience and outer realities. He believed that the therapeutic process would deepen understanding of emotions, thoughts, and behaviors that perpetuate difficulties, bring greater acceptance of the self, and improve psychological and social functioning, expanding capacities for love and work.

Freud introduced a range of approaches and techniques intended to help the patient suspend defenses, allowing derivatives of instinctual energies to emerge through free association and transference reactions to the therapist. He developed the method of free association—advising the patient to say what comes to mind in an accepting, non-judgmental manner—in an effort to circumvent the dynamics of defensive processes and activate conflictual experience in the clinical situation. In his conception of transference the patient re-experiences sensations, feelings, and thoughts he believed to originate in the dynamics of instinctual life.

Although Freud found that he could help patients recreate problematic feelings, thoughts, and actions in the therapeutic situation, he realized that insight itself did not necessarily bring about change. He came to believe that varying degrees of resistance are inevitable as we work toward growth, explaining:

> The resistance accompanies the treatment step by step. Every single association, every act of the person under treatment must reckon with the resistance and represents a compromise between the forces that are striving toward recovery and the opposing ones.
>
> (1912/1958, p. 103)

In introducing the principle of "working through" in his seminal paper on technique, "Remembering, repeating, and working through," Freud emphasizes that the therapist and patient must be prepared to engage recurring emotions, wishes, conflicts, defenses, and transference reactions as they emerge in different forms (1914/1958). Ongoing exploration and formulation of unconscious experience, resistance, and transference states deepen understanding of underlying motivations and conflicts, fostering integrations of neural networks and life experience. Carefully focused observation, challenge, and interpretation convey the clinician's efforts to grasp potential meanings hidden in the manifest content of words and the functions of behavior that operate out of awareness, deepening insight and understanding, helping the patient to re-appropriate aspects of self that have been repressed or repudiated. Acceptance and integration of dissociated sensations, feelings, and thoughts foster change and growth, strengthening the sense of self and identity, ego functions, and coping capacities.

As we have seen in earlier accounts of neural development, researchers assume that the repeated activation and processing of sensation, emotion, imagery, cognition, and behavior facilitates neural integration in accord with the principles of Hebbian learning or long-term potentiation (see Chapter 2). From the perspective of contemporary neuroscience, Freud introduced a range of therapeutic methods that allow us to explore the discontinuities and dissociations of neural networks encompassed in conscious and unconscious domains of experience, strengthening the development, integration, and regulation of the core structures and functions of the brain.

Jung and Analytical Psychology

Jung worked to bridge biological, psychological, and social domains of understanding in his formulations of personality and psychopathology, and he drew on the philosophical pragmatism of William James in his approach to theory, research, and practice, emphasizing "the extraordinary diversity of individual life" that we cannot "fit into any scheme... I have always felt the need for a conspectus of many viewpoints," he writes, "giving divergent opinions their view;" otherwise we are "doing violence to our own empirical material" (1929/1975, p. 36). Like James, he was critical of reductive versions of materialism that dismissed the value of subjective experience and personal meaning, seeking to join scientific and humanistic realms of understanding.

He completed medical school at the University of Zurich and trained in psychiatry at the Burgholzli clinic, where he worked as an assistant to Eugen Bleuler, known for having introduced the terms "schizophrenia" and "autism." Like Freud, Jung was influenced by Charcot's work and studied with his collaborator, Pierre Janet, at the Saltpetriere hospital, embracing the new field of dynamic psychiatry. Jung carried out research on unconscious processes over the course of his training at the Burgholzli, conducting word association experiments that would provide empirical foundations for his emerging formulations of the self and the dynamics of inner life.

He read *The interpretation of dreams* in 1900 and returned to the account three years later, sending Freud reports of his research on unconscious phenomena. They began corresponding in 1906; in time, Freud invited Jung to join his psychoanalytic study group. In 1909 Freud and Jung traveled to the United States, where they gave a series of lectures for the 20th anniversary celebration of the founding of Clark University in Worcester, Massachusetts. In the course of the visit they met William James. While Freud and James found themselves uneasy with one another—James describing Freud as fixed and rigid—Jung came to think of James as an exemplar, embracing his pragmatic philosophy.

Jung increasingly found Freud's thinking reductive and mechanistic, believing that he placed too much emphasis on sexuality as a motivating force in human life. While Freud saw the unconscious largely as the domain of instinctual life that precipitates conflict and symptoms, Jung proposed that the sexual instinct is but one aspect of human experience and regarded the unconscious region of the mind as a potential source of growth and creativity. Following his break with Freud in 1913, Jung initiated a deep exploration of his own experience that he recounts in his autobiography, *Memories, dreams, reflections* (1961). He began to formulate concepts and methods that would shape the development of his school of thought, known as analytical psychology, enlarging ways of understanding self, relational life, and the interactive field of psychotherapy. He came to believe that the search for wholeness and the integration of personality—what he described as the process of individuation—is the cardinal motivation in human development, and it shaped his conceptions of maturation across the course of life.

In fashioning his depth psychology Jung describes core structures of the personality thought to mediate the dynamics of psychic life. The psyche, like the body, is a self-regulating system. He conceives of the ego as the center of consciousness, encompassing our experience of emotions, thoughts, images, and memories, preserving cohesion and coherence in sense of self and identity. The executive functions of the ego facilitate efforts to negotiate inner experience and the outer realities of everyday life. He introduces the term persona to describe the functions of the public self, shaped by convention and tradition, facilitating efforts to carry out various roles.

The personal unconscious encompasses experiences that have been repressed, dissociated, forgotten, or ignored; it also holds experiences that we fail to register in conscious awareness, carried in what we now understand as implicit memory. The contents of the personal unconscious are potentially accessible to awareness through exploration and processing of experience.

Jung thinks of the collective unconscious as the source of memory traces inherited from the ancestral past encompassing the history of humans as a species, the cumulative outcome of repeated experience over many generations. The brain, he proposes,

> is inherited from its ancestors; it is the deposit of the psychic functioning of the whole human race… In the brain the instincts are preformed, and so are the primordial images which have always been the basis of man's thinking—the whole treasure house of mythological motifs.
>
> (1928/1978, pp. 310–311)

He introduced the concept of the archetype to describe the structural elements of the collective unconscious (Jung 1954/1968). The archetype, bridging the realms of body and mind, is an inherited part of the psyche that generates patterns of imagery and behavior. Jung distinguishes the "archetype as such" from the "archetype as image" as follows:

> By this I do not mean the existing form of the motif but its preconscious, invisible "ground plan." This might be compared to the crystal lattice that is preformed in the crystalline solution. It should not be confused with the variously structured axial system of the individual crystal.
>
> (Jung, 1928/1978, p. 311)

The tradition of Platonic thought, Kant's a priori categories of perception (see Chapter 7), and Schopenhauer's notion of prototypes prefigure Jung's formulations of the archetype, and the concept of innate psychological structure emerges later in the fields of evolutionary biology and behavioral genetics. Tradition and cultural life shape various expressions of archetypal elements.

Jung introduced the concept of the shadow to represent the negative elements of personality that we come to find personally or socially unacceptable—in his definition, "the thing a person has no wish to be" (1946/1975, p. 262). He emphasizes, however, that the shadow potentially carries generative elements that sponsor change and growth as we bring experience into consciousness.

Jung joins archetypal and personal realms of experience in his formulations of the complex, grounded in his empirical research on the dynamics of the unconscious. We can think of the complex as an admixture of sensations, emotions, images, and thoughts that operate out of awareness and influence behavior when activated in particular situations; from the perspective of contemporary neuroscience, we understand complexes as networks of association that originate in core constituents of "psychophysiology" (archetypal elements) and in the concrete particularity of individual experience over the course of development (personal elements). Complexes carry the potential to precipitate splits between conscious and unconscious domains of experience, fragmenting the self and constricting ways of being, relating, and living. Following traumatic experience they may operate autonomously as "splinter-psyches," he proposed, as if they have a consciousness of their own, perpetuating vicious circles of feeling, thought, and action.

Jung describes two fundamental orientations of personality in his formulations of psychological types, the "attitude types" of introversion and extraversion. The extraverted attitude orients the individual to the outer, objective world of activity. The introverted attitude orients the individual to the inner, subjective realm of experience. Both attitudes are present in the personality, Jung proposes, but one is more conscious and dominant. He conceptualizes four modes of functioning that characterize the ways in which we negotiate experience and process information: thinking, feeling, sensing, and intuiting. Thinking encompasses cognitive efforts to comprehend the nature of experience, including analysis, abstraction, generalization, reason, and judgment. Feeling emphasizes the subjective value of experience. Sensing is the perceptual or reality function, focused on concrete particulars. Intuition is a mode of perception mediated by unconscious processes and context. From the perspective of contemporary neuroscience, Jung describes fundamental differences in the processing functions of the right and left hemispheres of the brain. The left hemisphere is instrumental in thinking and sensing functions, while the right hemisphere is dominant in feeling and intuiting functions.

As Jung elaborated his conceptions of individuation he shifted the focus of attention from Freud's formulations of the ego—closely associated with the conscious, analytical, language-based functions of the left hemisphere—to the unconscious, emotional, non-verbal domains of the right hemisphere, now understood as the source of the bodily-based self system. As noted in Chapter 2, converging lines of study in developmental psychology and interpersonal neurobiology link the functions of the right hemisphere to the emergence of the corporeal and emotional sense of self, governing capacities for regulation of sensation and emotion, empathy, mentalization, and inter-subjectivity (Schore, 2019a, 2019b; see Wilkinson, 2006, 2015, for expanded accounts of developmental neuroscience and analytical psychology).

Although Jung recognizes the crucial role of the ego in coping and adaptation, he regards the self as the fundamental organizing principle of personality, regulating the dynamics of psychic life. The self is the core of the personality in its actual and potential forms. In his developmental schema, the self originates in an inborn dynamic structure integrating the core constituents of brain and mind. Jung proposed that the symbols of the self originate in the depths of the body and came to think of the self as the regulating system that governs maturation across the course of life. He writes: "The self is not only the centre, but also the whole circumference which embraces both conscious and unconscious; it is the centre of this totality, just as the ego is the centre of the conscious mind" (Jung 1946/1977, p. 41). The development of the self is shaped by emerging challenges, concerns, values, and goals; as such it is purposive or teleological. He describes the transcendent function as the maturational force that regulates ongoing efforts to integrate different elements of the personality, process unconscious constituents of the psyche and life experience, and work toward wholeness or individuation of self (for expanded accounts see Jung, 1934/1978; 1944/1993).

Jung's conceptions of the self prefigure orienting perspectives that have come to shape understanding in contemporary neuroscience, emphasizing the need to take account of the core structures and functions of the brain and the phenomenal world of the mind in accord with pragmatic formulations of "non-reductive materialism" outlined in Chapter 3. The human sciences must encompass "the *physical* and the *psychic*," he emphasizes, cautioning that "psychology does this only in so far as it is *psychophysiology*" (1946/1977 p. 87; italics added).

In line with Jung's formulations, Antonio Damasio describes a "preconscious biological precedent," the "protoself," that serves as the foundation for the emergence of the "core self." In his account of development, "Body and brain bond...the body is best conceived as the rock on which the protoself is built, while the protoself is the pivot around which the conscious mind turns" (2010, p. 21). Drawing on Jung's developmental model and recent research in neuroscience, Jaak Panksepp, Antonio Alcaro, and Stefano Carta have linked brain activity within subcortical structures to the emergence of prototypical affective states believed to influence the organization of personality, consciousness, and behavior (Alcaro, Carta & Panksepp, 2017). In accord with Jung's emphasis on the plurality of the psyche, Joseph LeDoux proposes that different domains of experience reflect the functions of different brain systems. While explicit memory is mediated by a single system, he observes, a variety of brain systems store information implicitly, "allowing for many aspects of self to coexist" (2002, p. 31). Like Jung, LeDoux understands the self as "the totality of what an organism is physically, biologically, psychologically, socially, and culturally" (2002, p 31).

Therapeutic Action

The fundamental aim of the therapeutic endeavor, from the perspective of analytical psychology, is to reinstate the maturational process that governs the dynamics of individuation—the psychic equilibrating force—and to integrate elements of the personality that have been split, dissociated, or unrealized. Conceptions of neural development, integration, and regulation described in Chapter 3 parallel this formulation of therapeutic action.

Jung took a pragmatic approach to psychotherapy, as noted, and he remained uneasy with efforts to reduce the therapeutic process to basic procedures or techniques. He embraced a pluralist outlook, emphasizing the concrete outcomes of ideas. "I have taken as my guiding principle William James' pragmatic rule: 'you must bring out of each word its practical cash value, set it at work within the stream of your experience'" (Jung, 1912/1976, p. 86).

He challenged psychotherapists to focus on the patient as an individual and to remain open and flexible in accord with the values of clinical pragmatism, considering different ways of working in light of our understanding of what is the matter, personality and temperament, stage in life, capacities and skills, and therapeutic outcomes. As he explains in his account of "The aims of psychotherapy," he allows "pure experience" and practical outcomes to shape the course of help and care, cautioning: "The shoe that fits one person pinches another; there is no universal recipe for living" (Jung, 1929/1975, p. 41).

He describes the ways in which efforts to manage trauma through dissociation can precipitate splits between conscious and unconscious realms of experience: "As a result of some psychic upheaval," he writes, "whole tracts of our being can plunge back into the unconscious and vanish from the surface for years and decades… disturbances caused by affects are known technically as phenomena of dissociation, and are indicative of a psychic split" (Jung, 1934/1978, pp. 138–139).

If problems in living and symptoms reflect signs of underlying trauma, he proposes, they also provide points of entry into less conscious realms of experience that carry the potential to bring about change and growth.

He explores the ways in which dreams and images deepen understanding of self and life experience, and dream analysis remains a defining feature of classical Jungian practice. In the reductive approach, the clinician and patient explore dream content in light of past experience, exploring, for example, the dynamics of early development, family life, and traumatic events. In the synthetic or constructive approach the patient and therapist focus on future possibilities, exploring dream content in light of symbolic meanings, emerging concerns, and efforts to realize potential in the individuation of the self.

He attempts to override neurotic patterns of behavior and engage unconscious domains of experience through his method of active imagination. As he describes it, the patient engages in dialogue with figures of the unconscious as they have emerged in dream images or in the conscious process of reflection and imagination. Dream analysis and active imagination carry the potential to provide access to the deeper healing influence of the psyche.

Jung anticipates fundamental developments in the contemporary relational paradigm, emphasizing the crucial role of the therapeutic alliance and inter-active experience in the two-person field. He describes the ways in which conscious and unconscious elements of the patient and therapist influence interaction over the course of the therapeutic process. In doing so he pre-figures reciprocal conceptions of transference and countertransference, and introduces ways of understanding interactive processes that foreshadow accounts of right-brain forms of communication described in Chapter 2.

He views transference and countertransference states as crucial sources of experience that deepen understanding of trauma, the dynamics of psychic func-tioning, and problems in living. He considers the ways in which earlier relation-ships and archetypal elements influence reactions, distinguishing the "personal" and the "archetypal" transference. The personal transference is shaped by pat-terns of expectation originating in earlier relational life; the patient recreates the experience of others through projection or selective perception of particular features of the therapist that correspond to earlier relationships. The archetypal transference originates in the dynamics of the collective unconscious rather than in the interpersonal experience of the patient (see Jung, 1946/1975; 1977).

Whereas Freud believed that countertransference reactions originate in the unconscious dynamics of the clinician, potentially compromising the therapeutic process, Jung regards the subjective experience of the practitioner as a "highly important organ of information" (1931/1975, p. 71). In accord with the values of clinical pragmatism, he emphasizes the mutuality of the therapeutic relationship and believes that the process carries the potential to transform the patient and the clinician as they engage the authenticity and authority of their experience. "For two personalities to meet is like mixing two different chemical substances: if there is any combination at all, both are transformed" (1931/1975, p. 71).

Over the course of his work Jung engaged essential concerns that converge with the principles of clinical pragmatism, joining scientific and humanistic domains of understanding, and emphasizing the individuality and subjectivity of the person; notions of agency and intention; the crucial role of the ther-apeutic relationship, collaboration, and dialogue; the co-creation of narrative and meaning; experiential learning; and inherent capacities for change, growth, and realization of potential in the ongoing individuation of the self. In doing so, as we will see in the following chapter, he anticipates fundamental devel-opments in the evolution of the psychoanalytic paradigm, prefiguring explora-tions of subjectivity, self, and relational life.

References

Alcaro, A., Carta, S. & Panksepp, J. (2017). The affective core of the self: A neuro-archetypal perspective on the foundations of human (and animal) subjectivity. *Fron-tiers in Psychology*, 8, 1424.

Blagys, M. & Hilsenroth, M. (2000). Distinctive activities of short-term psychodynamic-interpersonal psychotherapy: A review of the comparative psychotherapy process literature. *Clinical Psychology: Science and Practice*, 7 (2), 167–188.

Borden, W. (1999). Pluralism, pragmatism, and the therapeutic endeavor in brief dynamic treatment, in W. Borden (Ed.), *Comparative approaches in brief dynamic psychotherapy* (pp. 7–43). New York and London: Haworth Press.

Borden, W. (2000). The relational paradigm in contemporary psychoanalysis: Toward a psychodynamically-informed social work perspective. *Social Service Review*, 74(3), 352–379.

Borden, W. (2009). *Contemporary psychodynamic theory and practice: Toward a critical pluralism*. New York: Oxford University Press.

Borden, W. (2010). Taking multiplicity seriously: Pluralism, pragmatism, and integrative perspectives in social work practice, in W. Borden (Ed.), *Reshaping theory in contemporary social work* (pp. 3–28). New York: Columbia University Press.

Borden, W. & Clark, J. (2012). Contemporary psychodynamic theory, research, and practice: Implications for evidence-based practice, in T. Rzepnicki, S. McCracken & H. Briggs (Eds.), *From task-centered social work to evidence-based and integrative practice* (pp. 65–87). New York: Oxford University Press.

Brendel, D. (2006). *Healing psychiatry: Bridging the science/humanism divide*. Cambridge, MA: MIT Press.

Breuer, J. & Freud, S. (1893–1895/1955). Studies in hysteria, in J. Strachey (Ed. & Trans.), *The standard edition of the complete psychological works of Sigmund Freud*, Vol. 2 (pp. 1–305). London: Hogarth Press.

Curtis, R. (2020). Relational psychoanalytic/psychodynamic psychotherapy, in S. Messer & N. Kaslow (Eds.), *Essential psychotherapies* (pp. 71–108). New York: Guilford.

Damasio, A. (2010). *Self comes to mind*. New York: Pantheon.

Fonagy, P., Gergely, G., Jurist, E. L. & Target, M. (2018). *Affect regulation, mentalization and the development of the self*. London: Taylor & Francis.

Fonagy, P., Roth, A. & Higgitt, A. (2005). Psychodynamic psychotherapies: Evidence-based practice and clinical wisdom. *Bulletin of the Menninger Clinic*, 69 (1), 1–58.

Freud, S. (1890/1966). Psychical (or mental) treatment, in J. Strachey (Ed. and Trans.), *The standard edition of the complete psychological work of Sigmund Freud*, Vol. 7 (pp. 281–302).

Freud, S. (1893/1959). Some points in a comparative study of organic and hysterical paralyses, in E. Jones (Ed.), *Collected papers*, Vol. 1 (pp. 42–58). New York: Basic.

Freud, S. (1895/1966). Project for a scientific psychology, in J. Strachey (Ed. & Trans.), *The standard edition of the complete psychological work of Sigmund Freud*, Vol. 1 (pp. 281–392). London: Hogarth Press.

Freud, S. (1900/1953). The interpretation of dreams, in J. Strachey (Ed. & Trans.), *The standard edition of the complete psychological works of Sigmund Freud*, Vols. 4 & 5 (pp. 1–626). London: Hogarth Press.

Freud, S. (1912/1958). The dynamics of transference, in J. Strachey (Ed. and Trans.), *The standard edition of the complete psychological work of Sigmund Freud*, Vol. 12 (pp. 97–108). London: Hogarth Press.

Freud, S. (1914/1958). Remembering, repeating, and working-through, in J. Strachey (Ed. & Trans.), *Standard edition of the complete psychological works of Sigmund Freud*, Vol. 12 (pp. 145–157). London: Hogarth Press.

Freud, S. (1923/1961). The ego and the id, in J. Strachey (Ed. & Trans.), *The stan-dard edition of the complete psychological works of Sigmund Freud*, Vol 10 (pp. 2–66). London: Hogarth Press.

Freud, S. (1925/1989). An autobiographical study, in S. Freud, *The standard edition of the complete psychological works of Sigmund Freud*. New York: Norton.

Gibbons, M., Crits-Christoph, P. & Hearon, B. (2008). The empirical status of psychodynamic therapies. *Annual Review of Clinical Psychology*, 4, 93–108.

Glass, R. M. (2008). Psychodynamic psychotherapy and research evidence: Bambi survives Godzilla? *Journal of the American Medical Association*, 300 (13), 1587–1589.

Greenberg, J. & Mitchell, S. (1983). *Object relations in psychoanalysis*. Cambridge, MA: Harvard University Press.

Jung, C. G. (1912/1976). The theory of psychoanalysis, in H. Read, M. Fordham, G. Adler & W. McGuire (Eds.), *Collected Works of C. G. Jung*, Vol. 4 (pp. 85–226). Princeton, NJ: Princeton University Press.

Jung, C. G. (1928/1978). The psychological foundations of the belief in spirits, in H. Read, M. Fordham, G. Adler & W. McGuire (Eds.), *The collected works of C. G. Jung*, Vol. 8 (pp. 301–337). Princeton, NJ: Princeton University Press.

Jung, C. G. (1929/1975). The aims of psychotherapy, in H. Read, M. Fordham, G. Adler & W. McGuire (Eds.), *Collected works of C. G. Jung*, Vol. 16, p. 36–52). Princeton, NJ: Princeton University Press.

Jung, C. G. (1931/1975). Problems of modern psychotherapy, in H. Read, M. Fordham, G. Adler & W. McGuire (Eds.), *Collected works of C. G. Jung*, Vol. 16 (pp. 53–75). Princeton, NJ: Princeton University Press.

Jung, C. G. (1934/1978). The meaning of psychology for modern man, in H. Read, M. Fordham, G. Adler & W. McGuire (Eds.), *Collected Works of C. G. Jung, Vol.* 10 (pp. 134–157). Princeton, NJ: Princeton University Press.

Jung, C. G. (1944/1993). Psychology and alchemy: Introduction, in H. Read, M. Fordham, G. Adler & W. McGuire (Eds.), *Collected works of C. G. Jung*, Vol. 12 (pp. 39–47). Princeton, NJ: Princeton University Press.

Jung, C. G. (1946/1975). The psychology of the transference, in H. Read, M. Fordham, G. Adler & W. McGuire (Eds.) *Collected works of C. G. Jung*, Vol. 16 (pp. 164–323). Princeton, NJ: Princeton University Press.

Jung, C. G. (1946/1977). Analytical psychology and education, in H. Read, M. Fordham, G. Adler & W. McGuire (Eds.), *Collected works of C. G. Jung*, Vol. 17 (pp. 63–133). Princeton, NJ: Princeton University Press.

Jung, C. G. (1954/1968). Archetypes of the collective unconscious, in H. Read, M. Fordham, G. Adler & W. McGuire (Eds.), *Collected works of C. G. Jung*, Vol. 9 (pp. 3–41). Princeton, NJ: Princeton University Press.

Jung, C. G. (1961). *Memories, dreams, reflections*. New York: Random House.

Jung, C. G. (1977). Analytical psychology and education, in H. Read, M. Fordham, G. Adler & W. McGuire (Eds.) *Collected works of C. G. Jung: The development of personality*, Vol. 17 (pp. 65–132). Princeton, NJ: Princeton University Press.

Kandel, E. (2012). *The age of insight*. New York: Farrar, Straus & Giroux.

Kandel, E. (2018). *The disordered mind*. New York: Farrar, Straus & Giroux.

LeDoux, J. (2002). *Synaptic self: How our brains become who we are*. New York: Viking Penguin.

Leichsenring, F. (2009). Psychodynamic psychotherapy: A review of efficacy and effectiveness studies, in R. A. Levy & S. J. Ablon (Eds.), *Handbook of evidence-based psychodynamic therapy* (pp. 3–27). New York: Humana Press.

Leichsenring, F. & Rabung, S. (2009). Effectiveness of long-term psychodynamic psychotherapy: A meta-analysis. *Journal of the American Medical Association*, 300 (13), 1587–1589.

Luborsky, L. & Barrett, M. (2006). The history and empirical status of key psychoanalytic concepts. *Annual Review of Clinical Psychology*, 2, 1–19.

Mitchell, S. (1988). *Relational concepts in psychoanalysis.* Cambridge, MA: Harvard University Press.

Pribram, K. & Gill, M. (1976). *Freud's 'project' reassessed.* New York: Basic.

Schore, A. (2019a) *The development of the unconscious mind.* New York: Norton.

Schore, A. (2019b). *Right brain psychotherapy.* New York: Norton.

Shedler, J. (2006). *That was then, this is now: An introduction to contemporary psychodynamic psychotherapy for the rest of us.* Retrieved from http://jonathanshedler.com/writings/ (accessed March 3, 2019).

Shedler, J. (2010). The efficacy of psychodynamic psychotherapy. *American Psychologist*, 65 (2), 18–109.

Shedler, J. (2015). Where is the evidence for evidence-based psychotherapy? *Journal of Psychological Therapies in Primary Care*, 4, 47–59.

Solms M. (2018a). The scientific standing of psychoanalysis. *British Journal of Psychiatry International*, 15, 5–8.

Solms, M. (2018b). The neurobiological underpinnings of psychoanalytic theory and therapy. *Frontiers in Behavioral Neuroscience*, 12, 294.

Sulloway, F. (1979). *Freud: Biologist of the mind: Beyond the psychoanalytic legend.* New York: Basic.

Weinberg, J. & Westen, D. (2001). Science and psychodynamics: From arguments about Freud to data. *Psychological Inquiry*, 12 (3), 129–132.

Westen, D. (1998). The scientific legacy of Sigmund Freud: Toward a psychodynamically-informed psychological science. *Psychological Bulletin*, 124 (3), 333–371.

Westen, D. & Gabbard, G. (2002a). Developments in cognitive neuroscience: Conflict, compromise, and connectionism. *Journal of the American Psychoanalytic Association*, 50, 53–90.

Westen, D. & Gabbard, G. (2002b). Developments in cognitive neuroscience: Implications for theories of transference. *Journal of the American Psychoanalytic Association*, 50, 99–134.

Westen, D., Novotny, C. M. & Thompson-Brenner, H. (2004). The empirical status of empirically supported psychotherapies: Assumptions, findings, and reporting in controlled clinical trials. *Psychological Bulletin*, 130 (4), 631–663.

Westen, D. (2005). Implications of research in cognitive neuroscience for psychodynamic psychotherapy, in G. Gabbard, J. Beck & J. Holmes (Eds.), *Oxford textbook of psychotherapy* (pp. 443–448). New York: Oxford University Press. Wilkinson, M. (2006). *Coming into mind: The mind-brain relationship: A Jungian clinical perspective.* London: Routledge.

Wilkinson, M. (2015). Mind, brain and body. *Journal of Analytical Psychology*, 62 (4), 526–543.

5   The Psychodynamic Paradigm
Relational Perspectives

...they are not all exploring elephants. Some may be grappling with giraffes. To try to contain the same reports within one framework may lead to strange hybrids: four stout legs; a long, graceful neck; four thin legs; a long trunk; and so on.

–Stephen Mitchell

Although Freud's drive psychology served as the orienting paradigm in classical psychoanalytic thought through the first half of the 20th century, a growing number of thinkers challenged his vision of human nature and therapeutic action, introducing alternative perspectives that would broaden the scope of understanding and practice. In this chapter I trace the emergence of relational perspectives in Europe and North America, showing how thinkers reformulated ways of understanding mind and self, relationship and social life, vulnerability and psychopathology, health and well-being, and the dynamics of therapeutic action. I describe the defining features of three schools of thought, broadly categorized as object relations psychology, interpersonal psychoanalysis, and self psychology, that have shaped the relational paradigm in contemporary psychoanalysis. I review the orienting perspectives of the relational model and outline basic assumptions, core concepts, and essential concerns that guide formulations of therapeutic action, change, and growth. In doing so I consider points of connection with recent developments in the science of mind and the basic principles and values of clinical pragmatism.

Origins

Like Jung, Alfred Adler, Otto Rank, and Sandor Ferenczi—originally members of Freud's inner circle—also came to challenge the core propositions of classical drive psychology. They increasingly emphasized the role of relational life, social surrounds, and culture in fashioning their accounts of personality development, vulnerability, and problems in living. They found the fundamental methods of classical psychoanalysis limiting and introduced more active forms of intervention focused on immediate concerns, emphasizing the crucial functions of collaboration, interpersonal interaction, and experiential learning. The following account, expanding earlier writings on the history of psychoanalysis, reviews the contributions of early revisionist thinkers who shaped the emergence of relational perspectives (Borden, 1999, 2000 2009, 2018; Borden & Clark, 2012).

Although Adler did not codify his theories in a systematic manner, as Freud had, he pursued fundamental concerns and themes over the course of his practice, introducing a relational perspective that would provide a radical alternative to drive psychology. He understood people as "social beings," deeply connected and interdependent, and he focused on the fundamental role of relationship, community, and social life in formulating his conceptions of development, resilience, and the common good. He elaborated a holistic conception of personality that emphasized the unity of body and mind, agency and free will, the search for meaning, and social responsibility (Adler, 1927/1992). He increasingly engaged moral and ethical concerns as he shaped his point of view and elaborated a psychology of values that would influence the humanistic perspectives of Abraham Maslow and Carl Rogers (see Chapter 8).

Over the course of development, Adler proposed in his accounts of social interest, we come to feel a deep sense of connection with humankind, recognizing our interconnectedness and interdependence, realizing that the welfare of any one individual depends on the well-being of the larger community. Constructive relationships and sustaining communities are characterized by mutual respect, attunement and empathy, trust, cooperation, and personal equality (Adler, 1927/1992).

Adler emphasized the importance of dialogue, narrative, and the co-creation of meaning in his conceptions of therapeutic action, anticipating the emergence of constructivist approaches in the cognitive paradigm (see Chapter 7). As a practitioner he preferred active and briefer forms of intervention, employing what we would now describe as cognitive, behavioral, educational, and task-centered methods, emphasizing experiential learning and the practical outcomes of help and care. As an advocate of social justice he initiated reform in the fields of education, social welfare, and public health. He came to encompass family, group, and community perspectives in integrative models of practice.

Rank, known for his scholarship in art, literature, philosophy, and mythology, focused on existential concerns as he fashioned his humanistic models of personality. He centered on the dynamics of autonomy, dependency, and individuation in developing his relational perspective, introducing notions of agency, will, responsibility, and action in his formulations of therapeutic action, change, and growth (Rank, 1936). He came to think of the individual as an initiator of action and interpreter of meaning, emphasizing conscious motives and goals rather than unconscious realms of experience, focusing on present circumstances and on anticipated future rather than past events.

He assumed that maladaptive patterns of functioning established over the course of relational life would emerge in the therapeutic process, providing in-vivo occasions to work through earlier experience and strengthen capacities to act and negotiate problems in living. In accord with Dewey's pragmatic thought, he saw the dynamics of experiential learning as fundamental mechanisms of change and growth. His ideas shaped the development of the field of brief psychotherapy and basic principles of intervention in the collective wisdom of social work practice. More broadly, his emphasis on relationship, will, and creativity influenced a range of existential thinkers in humanistic psychology, notably Rollo May and Irvin Yalom (see Chapter 8).

Like Adler, Ferenczi broadened the scope of the psychoanalytic paradigm, emphasizing the ways in which social, cultural, political, and economic conditions perpetuate restrictions of opportunity and problems in living. He founded a free clinic in Budapest, focusing his practice on marginalized and oppressed groups. He increasingly centered on the dynamics of family life and the concrete realities of actual experience in the outer world as he formulated his conceptions of vulnerability and trauma. He related a range of problems in functioning to lapses in earlier care, emphasizing the traumatic effects of empathic failings and deprivation in relational life.

Ferenczi recognized the crucial importance of the therapeutic alliance and the sustaining functions of the practitioner's attunement, empathy, and responsiveness, viewing the relationship as a collaborative, mutually supportive partnership. He proposed that enactments, transference states, and countertransference reactions provide points of entry into the dynamics of earlier experience, creating in-vivo occasions to rework patterns of behavior and establish new ways of being and relating. He departed from the neutral stance that Freudians had advocated and introduced the "rule of empathy" as a fundamental principle of psychotherapy, coming to see emotion as the transformative element of change and growth (Ferenczi, 1932/1949). He outlined revisions of analytic technique in *The development of psychoanalysis* (1924), co-authored with Rank. He continued to expand concepts of therapeutic action in his later work, integrating behavioral strategies and relaxation techniques, seeking to reduce the length of treatment and improve outcomes, anticipating fundamental concerns that would shape the field of brief psychotherapy (Borden, 1999).

Although the contributions of these early thinkers remain absent or marginal in most accounts of the psychodynamic paradigm, they anticipate essential concerns in the emergence of relational understanding and prefigure the growing emphasis on active, integrative forms of therapy in contemporary practice.

The collective experience of trauma, loss, and mourning in Great Britain after World War I changed the course of psychoanalytic understanding and therapeutic practice through the 1920s. A diverse group of practitioners associated with the Tavistock Clinic in London, drawing on the work of Jung, Adler, and Ferenczi, increasingly focused on the dynamics of relational life as they cared for patients following the widespread experience of separation, loss, and grief. Ian Suttie, one of the most creative thinkers of the group, proposed that innate needs for relationship and love are the fundamental motivations of personality development, focusing on the generative functions of relationship and community life and the role of "social interest" in his notions of health, well-being, and the common good (Suttie, 1935). He argued that problems in living are shaped more by family dynamics, stressful circumstances, and social and cultural conditions than by universal biological forces. Like Ferenczi, he emphasized the healing functions of the therapeutic relationship, the role of emotion, and the dynamics of interactive experience in change and growth.

The generation of thinkers that followed, including Melanie Klein, W. R. D. Fairbairn, Donald W. Winnicott, and John Bowlby, continued to carry out radical revisions of psychoanalytic thinking that would shape relational perspectives throughout the second half of the 20th century.

Working in the Freudian tradition, Klein preserved classical notions of drive and emphasized the dynamics of fantasy life in her conceptions of the self. Over the course of her work, however, she introduced concepts of internal representation ("internal objects"), defensive processes ("splitting" and "projective identification"), and self-organization that provided crucial points of departure for Fairbairn, Winnicott, and Bowlby as they elaborated their relational perspectives. While many thinkers criticize Klein for her failure to consider the role of interpersonal experience, social conditions, and cultural factors in her models of personality development, she provided a crucial bridge to the object relations tradition, emerging as a seminal figure in the transition from drive to relational perspectives.

Like Suttie, Fairbairn placed relationship at the center of human life, elaborating models of development that have come to serve as the foundation for contemporary object relations perspectives. We are inherently oriented to others at birth, he proposed, and fundamental needs for contact and relationship shape behavior throughout life (Fairbairn, 1952). In his developmental schema, the self is structured through the internalization and representation of interpersonal experience as schemas or models of relational life. He documents the ways in which lapses in care, neglect, abuse, and trauma compromise the course of development and perpetuate problems in living. Like Ferenczi, he emphasizes the crucial role of the therapeutic alliance and the dynamics of enactment, transference states, and interactive experience in working through the failings of relational life.

Winnicott centered on the emergence of the self as he formulated his accounts of development, emphasizing the ways in which the constancy of care in the holding environment of infancy and early childhood fosters maturation, health, and well-being. "There is no such thing as a baby," Winnicott wrote, focusing on the intersubjective dynamics of care. "One sees a nursing couple" (1952/1975, p. 99). He proposed that we are born with an inherent motivation to actualize the "true self" and described the dynamics of the "maturational process" that governs the "drive towards integration" and the development of the individual (Winnicot, 1963/1965, p. 239; see Chapters 3 and 9, this volume). He described three processes that mediate the development of the self—"integration," "personalization," and "object relating"—and corresponding caretaking provisions that foster maturation of core structures, psyche-soma integration, and capacities to negotiate relational life: "holding," "handling," and "object relating" (for expanded review of developmental concepts see Borden, 2009, 2018). Although lapses and fail-ings in care may undermine the integrative functions of the maturational process, Winnicott believed that we continue to search for conditions that carry the potential to reinstate the course of development. He increasingly centered on subjective experience in elaborating his developmental psychol-ogy, most fully realized in his conceptions of embodiment and the "true self," emphasizing our capacities for aliveness, inner coherence, authenticity, agency, personal meaning, creativity, and play.

In accord with the values and sensibilities of the Independent Tradition in the British Psycho-Analytic Society, Winnicott was committed to a pragmatist ethics in his approach to help and care, as noted in the Introduction. He refused to codify his ideas in a grand theory, explaining: "…my mind doesn't work that way… I gather this and that, here and there, settle down to clinical experience…" (1945/1975, p. 145). He rejected standard models of psycho-analysis and remained steadfast in his efforts to carry out "experiments in adapting to need," using whatever ideas and methods offered purchase in light of the possibilities and constraints of the given case (Winnicott, 1971; see Chapter 9 this volume).

Bowlby joined the orienting perspectives of Darwinian thought, develop-mental biology, ethology, infant observation research, and dynamic systems theory as he formed his conceptions of attachment, emphasizing close analy-sis of behavior, deepening our understanding of the bond between children and parents. He argued that the fundamental need to establish contact and connection has adaptive roots in biological survival; relational life, he believed, is grounded in the genetics and physiology of human development. Drawing on cognitive psychology, he proposed that we internalize and represent fundamental elements of relational experience as mental structures, forming schemas or "working models" of self and others that guide ways of processing information and patterns of interpersonal behavior; in this sense his formulations converge with the basic proposals of Fairbairn and object relations psychology, described in the following section. He emphasized the ways in which the clinician provides a "secure base" as the patient processes earlier experiences of separation, trauma, and loss, reworking inner models of relational life that perpetuate problems in living, attending to transference states and particular patterns of behavior that emerge over the course of help and care (Bowlby, 1988).

Bowlby's work informed the development of observational research that documented the ways in which infants actively seek stimulation and promote attachment to primary figures who provide protection and support. Mary Ainsworth introduced the controlled setting of the "strange situation," demonstrating different kinds of attachment styles seen in a novel circumstance of controlled separation from the primary caretaking figure. Mary Main studied the dynamics of attachment across generations, exploring the relationship between a parent's early attachment experiences and the infant's attachment status. Converging lines of study in developmental psychology and the fields of neuroscience have continued to explore the role of interactive experience in the maturation of the brain and the emergence of the self, influencing patterns of adaptation across the course of life (for expanded reviews see Fonagy, 2001; Schore, 2019a, 2019b; Siegel, 2020; Sroufe, 2016).

Harry Stack Sullivan, Karen Horney, Clara Thompson, Frieda Fromm-Reichmann, and Eric Fromm shaped the emergence of interpersonal psycho-analysis in North America throughout the 1930s and 1940s, introducing social and cultural perspectives that enlarged conceptions of personality development, relational life, and therapeutic action.

Sullivan drew on American pragmatism and divergent thinkers in the Chicago school of social science, including George Herbert Mead, W. I. Thomas, and Edward Sapir, as he elaborated process-oriented models of personality and mind that centered on the dynamics of relational life and the social surround. Like Bowlby, he brought an empirical disposition to his work, attending to what we say and do in the "me-you" patterns of interactive experience. He focused on the concrete particulars of life as sensed and felt, the formative role of social interaction in understanding and problem-solving, and the practical outcomes of ideas. Moved by the example of Jane Addams, he set out to engage vulnerable, disenfranchised groups in help and care, focusing on real-life concerns, hoping to democratize psychotherapy.

In formulating his developmental psychology, Sullivan proposed that the experience of dependency and conditions of care through infancy and child-hood inevitably generate vulnerability, fear, and anxiety as we negotiate the possibilities and constraints of relational life in the social surround. Over the course of development, he theorized, we elaborate repetitive patterns of beha-vior in ongoing efforts to reduce fear and anxiety, increase security and satis-faction, and preserve connections with others (Sullivan, 1953). He described the dynamics of the "self system" that sanctions certain forms of behavior (the "good-me" self), prohibits other forms of behavior (the "bad me" self) and excludes from consciousness ways of being that are too threatening to imagine (the "not-me" self). He thought of the self-system as a filter for awareness, introducing the concept of "selective inattention" to describe unconscious refusals to register experience that intensifies fear and anxiety.

Sullivan challenged reductive taxonomies of psychopathology, preferring to speak of "dynamisms of difficulty" and "problems in living" in accord with the "one genus postulate" that he introduced in his case seminars: "we are all much more simply human than otherwise" (Sullivan, 1953, p. 32). His formulations of problems in living center on the ways in which defensive processes perpetuate maladaptive patterns of thought, feeling, and action. He viewed the clinician as a participant-observer in the therapeutic process, emphasizing the role of inter-personal interaction, active forms of intervention, and experiential learning in change and growth.

Horney enlarged conceptions of self and relational life through the 1940s and 1950s, exploring the ways in which the dynamics of family life and social and cultural conditions influence the course of development, gender identity, patterns of interpersonal behavior, and problems in living. In her formulations of neurosis, fear and anxiety constrict ways of being, relating, and living, limiting realization of potential. She elaborated interpersonal conceptions of defense and described "vicious circles" of thought, feeling, and action that perpetuate problems in living (Wachtel expands these formulations in his integrative model, described in Chapter 6).

As she developed her relational perspective she came to think of the defining feature of neurosis—"a special form of human development antithetical to human growth"—as alienation from the core self, originating in pathogenic conditions in the social surround (Horney, 1950, p. 13). "It is the process of abandoning the real self for an idealized one: of trying to actualize this pseudo-self instead of our given human potential..." (1950, p. 371). Abraham Maslow and Carl Rogers drew on her work in shaping their conceptions of humanistic psychology (see Chapter 8). In line with her developmental formulations, Horney emphasized mutual sources of recognition, empathy, and influence in the therapeutic relationship; emotion and intuition as modes of knowing; and the role of experiential learning as the patient challenges neurotic patterns of behavior and re-appropriates the authenticity and authority of self.

Heinz Kohut explored fundamental concerns in the realm of subjectivity as he shaped his psychology of the self in North America in the 1970s and 1980s, focusing on the sense of cohesion and coherence in states of being; the feeling of aliveness and vitality; capacities for agency and initiative; and the ways in which we generate experience that we register as real, meaningful, and distinctly our own. He centered on the fundamental need to establish a unitary, integrated sense of self and the crucial role of relational life in health, well-being, and optimal functioning. He focused on the ways in which the dynamics of mirroring and interactive experience foster the emergence of the self over the course of care, exploring the dyadic features of unconscious communication and regulation between the infant and caretakers, anticipating formulations of intersubjectivity. He introduced the concept of the "selfobject" in his developmental schema, defining the construct as an intrapsychic experience of a person, object, or activity that strengthens and sustains the self (Kohut, 1977). He proposed that the selfobject functions of caretakers are gradually internalized as self-functions, or inner psychic structure, through the process of "transmuting internalization," fostering the development of capacities for self-cohesion, self-regulation, and self-righting.

The fundamental aim of psychotherapy, from the perspective of self psychology, is to reinstate developmental processes that have been compromised by earlier lapses in care. The therapist's empathic attunement and responsiveness as a selfobject strengthen the integrity of the self. Kohut described three forms of selfobject transference—mirroring, idealizing, and twinship—that provide experiential opportunities for the restoration of the self. He emphasized the crucial role of "vicarious introspection" and "protracted empathic immersion" as the patient engages selfobject functions instrumental in healing, change, and growth (1971, p. 300).

Relational Schools of Thought

The writings of the foregoing thinkers, placing relationship at the center of human experience, shaped the development of three schools of thought in the psychodynamic paradigm, broadly described as object relations theories, interpersonal psychoanalysis, and self psychology. Although scholars did not attempt to establish overarching frameworks, they emphasized overlapping concerns and themes in their developmental formulations and therapeutic approaches. I briefly review orienting perspectives that have guided understanding and practice in each tradition, expanding earlier accounts of the psychoanalytic paradigm (Borden, 2009; see Borden & Clark, 2012, for a review of relational models, empirical research, and implications for evidence-based practice).

Object Relations Perspectives

Contemporary object relations perspectives, shaped by the developmental formulations of Ferenczi, Klein, Suttie, Fairbairn, and Bowlby, continue to center on the ways in which the dynamics of motivation, emotion, and cognition influence subjective states of self, perceptions of others, and patterns of interpersonal behavior. Clinical scholars propose that basic prototypes of connection, formed over the course of caretaking and early relational life, are structured as internalized representations of self and others. Although thinkers assume that core representations originate in the dynamics of interpersonal experience, they believe that inner models of relational life are also influenced by individual differences in constitution and temperament, regulatory functions, and unconscious fantasy processes. The dynamics of interoception and emotion, emerging needs, interpersonal interaction, and life circumstances are thought to influence the particular representations guiding perception and behavior at any given time. We experience others as we *perceive* them, not necessarily as they actually are (Wachtel, 2011).

Conceptions of vulnerability and psychopathology focus on the ways in which inner models of self and others influence perceptions of relational life, activate defensive processes, and perpetuate maladaptive patterns of behavior. Thinkers have reformulated Klein's accounts of "splitting" and "projective identification" from a relational point of view, expanding conceptions of defense. Models of therapeutic action center on the dynamics of interaction and experiential learning as patients process enactments, transference states, and countertransference reactions; reorganize maladaptive defenses; enlarge inner representations of self and others; and strengthen capacities to negotiate the course of relational life.

Object relations perspectives have guided empirical study of personality development, trauma, psychopathology, and therapeutic practice over the last three decades. Developmental lines of study have explored the dynamics of caretaking experience, patterns of attachment, interactive forms of communication and emotional regulation, and emerging capacities to negotiate relational life.

Research findings corroborate the assumption that infants are pre-adapted to form attachments and engage in complex forms of interaction with caretaking figures (Beebe & Lachmann, 2013; Fonagy, 2001; Fonagy & Target, 2007; Schore, 2019a, 2019b; Solms, 2018a, 2018b; Stern, 1985, 2004). Longitudinal studies document the ways in which attachment styles and dyadic caregiving systems influence development of personality organization, capacities to regulate emotion, interpersonal functioning, and patterns of coping and adaptation (see Fonagy, 2001; Fonagy & Target, 2007; Schore, 2019a, 2019b; Siegel, 2020; Solms, 2018a, 2018b; Sroufe, 2016; Sroufe, Egelund, Carlson & Collins, 2005).

Research on perception, learning, and memory in the field of cognitive neuroscience has provided considerable support for object relations formulations of unconscious mental processing and mental representations of self, others, and of relational life (Schore, 2019a; Solms, 2018a; Westen, 1998, 2005; Westen & Gabbard, 2002a, 2002b). Converging lines of study corroborate conceptions of transference, documenting the ways in which the dynamics of interpersonal interaction activate inner representations of self and others; motivational, emotional, and cognitive processes, and corresponding patterns of behavior (Gabbard & Westen, 2002a, 2002b; Schore, 2012, 2019a, 2019b; Solms, 2018a, 2018b).

Clinical researchers have explored the ways in which inner models of relational experience and patterns of social cognition precipitate problems in functioning associated with depression, acute stress reactions, post-traumatic stress disorders, personality disorders, and other forms of developmental psychopathology (see reviews by Blatt & Homan, 1992; Borden & Clark, 2012; Fonagy & Target, 2007; Luborsky & Barrett, 2006; Masling & Bornstein, 1994; Messer & Kaslow, 2020; Roth & Fonagy, 2005; Westen, 1998, 2005, 2007; Westen, Novotny & Thompson-Brenner, 2004).

Interpersonal Perspectives

Whereas object relations perspectives center on the role of internalization processes and mental representations of self and others, interpersonal approaches focus on overt patterns of behavior in the interactive fields of relational life, expanding the developmental models of Sullivan and Horney reviewed in the preceding section. Clinical scholars have continued to elaborate process-oriented conceptions of mind and self, exploring the ways in which the changing contexts of relational life influence subjective experience, the dynamics of defense, and patterns of behavior. Integrative thinkers assume that there is an isomorphic relationship between inner models of relational life and patterns of behavior in the outer world, viewing object relations and interpersonal approaches as complementary perspectives.

In working from an interpersonal perspective, the patient and therapist explore the dynamics of anxiety, defense, enactments, and maladaptive patterns of behavior as they emerge in the clinical situation, engaging opportunities for experiential learning that foster the development of relational capacities and interpersonal skills. As noted earlier, Sullivan views the clinician as a "participant-observer" in the interpersonal field of the therapeutic process. The concept of interpersonal complementarity is a basic principle of interpersonal theory: patterns of behavior tend to evoke particular types of reactions from others, which reinforce negative self-appraisals and expectations of others (Borden, 2009; Wachtel, 2008). Countertransference reactions emerge as role-responsive complements or counterparts to the patient's ways of being and relating. As we will see, Sullivan's formulations converge with concepts of therapeutic action in third-wave behavioral models of intervention, emphasizing the importance of experiential learning in change and growth (see Chapter 6).

The core concepts of interpersonal psychoanalysis have guided formulations of interactive experience in empirical studies of psychotherapy over the last three decades (see Benjamin, 1993; Curtis, 2020; Leichsenring, 2009; Levenson, 2017; Luborsky & Crits-Christoph, 1990; Strupp & Binder, 1984). Investigators have examined the relationship between social information processing and transference phenomena, documenting the dynamics of motivation, emotion, and cognition and the activation of "interpersonal scripts" or schemas that specify particular patterns of interpersonal behavior (see Shedler, 2010; Solms, 2018a, 2018b; Westen, 2005). Recent reviews of the literature document the effectiveness of interpersonal approaches for a range of conditions, including depression, anxiety disorders, post-traumatic stress disorder, and personality disorders (for reviews of empirical findings see Curtis, 2020; Gibbons, Crits-Christoph & Hearon, 2008; Leichsenring & Rabung 2009; Luborsky & Barrett, 2006; Roth & Fonagy, 2005; Shedler, 2010; Solms, 2018a, 2018b).

Self Psychology

Clinical scholars have continued to expand Kohut's formulations of development, psychopathology, and psychotherapy, exploring points of connection with object relations perspectives, interpersonal schools of thought, and conceptions of intersubjectivity. Thinkers center on the fundamental need to establish a unitary, integrated sense of self and the sustaining functions of relationship across the course of life. Developmental formulations describe the ways in which the empathic attunement, responsiveness, and provisions of caretakers or selfobjects foster the emergence of a cohesive sense of self. Researchers have documented the dynamics of synchrony, rupture, and interactive repair in attachment and relational life, theorizing that caretaking functions are internalized as psychic structure, facilitating efforts to regulate states of self. Failures in empathic responsiveness are believed to compromise the development of the self, leading to structural deficits and defensive patterns of behavior. Clinicians describe a range of problems in functioning associated with disorders of the self, including difficulties in preserving cohesion and continuity in subjective experience and sense of identity, regulating emotion, maintaining self-esteem and morale, negotiating interpersonal life, and pursuing meaningful goals and activities.

Following Kohut's reformulations of therapeutic action, clinicians focus on the critical functions of relational provisions believed to strengthen the self and regulate the dynamics of inner life. The therapist's empathic attunement and responsiveness as a selfobject foster the development of psychic structure through the process of "transmuting internalization," strengthening the integrity and regulatory functions of the self. For Kohut, health, well-being, and the good life depend on the "responsive selfobject milieu" (1984, p. 21).

Over the last three decades, converging lines of study have corroborated core concepts of development, exploring the ways in which infants and care-givers mutually influence states of self through interactive communication and regulation of emotion. Daniel Stern described four "domains of relatedness," influenced by constitution and temperament, innate maturational capacities, and the attunement and responsiveness of caretakers, that shape the emergence of the self (Stern, 1985, 2004). Beatrice Beebe and Frank Lachman documented the dynamics of ongoing regulation, rupture and repair, and heightened emotional moments over the course of their research (Beebe & Lachman, 2013). Allan Schore has drawn on core concepts from self psychology in elaborating neurobiological models of development, focusing on the experience-dependent maturation of the right brain, as discussed in Chapter 3 (2003a, 2003b, 2012, 2019a, 2019b). Longitudinal studies show that patterns of emotion, cognition, and behavior established in infancy and early childhood continue to shape the course of interpersonal functioning and adjustment in adulthood (Fonagy & Target, 2007; Siegel, 2020; Sroufe, 2016; Westen, 1998).

Schore has reformulated conceptions of trauma, post-traumatic stress disorder, and borderline personality organization, exploring the ways in which interactive experience over the course of psychotherapy influences the neurobiology of regulatory structures (Schore, 2019b). A large body of research on the core conditions of the therapeutic relationship and management of strain and rupture in the therapeutic alliance documents the crucial role of the practitioner's presence, empathic attunement, and responsiveness in determining the process and outcomes of treatment (see reviews by Curtis, 2020; Horvath, 2006; Roth & Fonagy, 2005; Schore, 2019a, 2019b; Wampold, 2015; Wolitzky, 2020).

The Relational Paradigm

The above perspectives emerged as independent schools of thought in Great Britain and North America over the second half of the 20th century, and there was surprisingly little dialogue or collaboration among the members of the different groups as they elaborated their developmental formulations and concepts of therapeutic action. Although all of them rejected drive psychology and emphasized the crucial role of relational life in human experience, they did not explore shared concerns or points of connection. Fairbairn and Sullivan, the principal architects of object relations psychology and interpersonal psychoanalysis, remained unaware of one another's contributions over the course of their work; Kohut failed to explore connections between his psychology of the self and the earlier writings of Suttie, Fairbairn, Winnicott, or Bowlby. In the early 1980s, however, clinical scholars began to carry out comparative studies of theoretical perspectives and clinical strategies, seeking to clarify the defining features and overlapping elements of the different approaches.

In their seminal work, *Object relations in psychoanalysis*, Jay Greenberg and Stephen Mitchell distinguished two competing paradigms that had shaped the development of psychoanalytic thought, broadly described as the drive model and the relational model (1983). They had originally used the term "relational" to bridge the British versions of object relations psychology and the American school of interpersonal psychoanalysis. In time, however, Mitchell expanded the scope of the relational perspective, encompassing emerging lines of study in self psychology and intersubjectivity, attachment research, social constructivism, narrative psychology, postmodern feminist thought, gender studies, and systems theory. He continued to carry out comparative studies of ideas and methods across the schools of thought, reformulating Freudian conceptions of constitutionality, embodiment, sexuality, aggression, and meaning from a relational perspective.

Mitchell joined the orienting perspectives of self psychology, object relations theory, and interpersonal psychoanalysis in developing an integrative framework, focusing on core domains of experience in his conception of the relational matrix: self-organization, internal representations of self and others and models of interaction; and patterns of behavior in the changing contexts of interpersonal life. As he showed in his accounts of clinical practice, the relational schools of thought focus our attention on overlapping realms of experience from different points of view, shaping complementary ways of understanding therapeutic action, change, and growth.

Over the course of his work he fashioned a conceptual synthesis that would serve as the foundation of relational psychoanalysis, emphasizing the practical utility of theories (Mitchell, 1988, 1993, 1997, 2000). In doing so he recognized crucial points of connection with the pragmatism of William James (see Mitchell & Harris, 2004). In framing the editorial philosophy of the international journal he founded, *Psychoanalytic Dialogues*, he proposed: "We need to regard differences in theoretical perspectives not as unfortunate deviations from accurate understanding but as fortunate expressions of the complex ways in which human experience can be organized" (Mitchell, 1991, p. 6). Some thinkers may be "exploring elephants," he wrote, while others may be "grappling with giraffes. To try to contain all reports within the same framework may lead to strange hybrids: four stout legs; a long, graceful neck; four tin legs; a long trunk; and so on" (1988, viii). In line with the principles of clinical pragmatism, he embraced theoretical pluralism and urged therapists to make use of ideas and methods from a range of perspectives as they carry out their practice, fashioning a personal synthesis in the concrete particularity of the clinical situation. Mitchell died unexpectedly in 2000, at the peak of his intellectual powers, having documented "the emergence of a tradition" (Mitchell & Aron, 1999).

The relational paradigm has continued to evolve over the last two decades, shaped by a divergent group of scholars, researchers, and practitioners, expanding conceptions of mind, self, identity, gender, race, sexuality, relationship, social life, trauma, and therapeutic action. Thinkers continue to explore the multiplicity and diversity of human experience, emphasizing the importance of open-ended dialogue across the fields of neuroscience, developmental psychology, philosophy, social thought, political theory, and the humanities (Barness, 2018). I briefly outline orienting perspectives, basic assumptions, and core concepts that guide understanding and practice across the relational paradigm, drawing on earlier accounts of the model (Borden, 2000, 2009; Borden & Clark, 2012; see Aron & Harris, 2011a, 2011b; Aron & Lechich, 2012; Curtis, 2020; for reviews of theoretical developments and clinical perspectives, see Harris, 2011; for accounts of relational psychoanalysis, gender, sexuality, race, class, ethnicity, and intersectionality, see Belkin & White, 2020).

Personality, Self, and Mind

Following the shift from Freud's drive psychology to the relational paradigm, clinical scholars have focused on the ways in which the dynamics of relational life shape the development of personality, self, and mind. From this perspective, the core constituents of human experience are not biological instincts as Freud had proposed but relations with others. The self is constituted and constructed in a relational matrix, and the focal concern is the interactive field of self, others, and relational life. Researchers emphasize fundamental needs for attachment and relationship across the course of life in elaborating conceptions of motivation and development.

From the perspective of self psychology, as we have seen, thinkers center on the sustaining functions of caretaking figures and the dynamics of interactive experience believed to foster the emergence of a cohesive sense of self. From the perspective of object relations theory, theorists consider the ways in which the internalization of interpersonal experience shapes the organization of the self and capacities for relatedness. As described earlier, thinkers assume that prototypes of connection, established in infancy and childhood, are structured in the form of internalized representations of self and others, mediating subjective states, perceptions of others, and patterns of interpersonal behavior. From the perspective of interpersonal psychoanalysis, thinkers conceive of personality as process, emphasizing the ways in which the course of relational life and the changing contexts of social surrounds shape subjective experience, the dynamics of defense, and patterns of behavior. Relational scholars speak of a "two-person psychology," emphasizing the intersubjective aspects of personality, self, and mind.

There is a dynamic organization to the ways in which we unconsciously register experience, shaped by the course of relational life. Clinical scholars have expanded conceptions of unconscious structures and experience in the relational paradigm, distinguishing three forms of unconsciousness that Robert Stolorow and George Atwood had introduced in their original formulations of intersubjectivity: the pre-reflective unconscious, encompassing organizing principles that shape experience and meaning; the dynamic unconscious, encompassing experiences that were denied articulation because they were perceived as threatening conditions of care in relational life; and the unvalidated unconscious, encompassing experiences that could not be validated because they never evoked the validating responses from the surround (Stolorow & Atwood, 1992). Christopher Bollas described the experience of the "unthought known" in his elaborations of the Freudian unconscious (1989). Interpersonal thinkers have emphasized the dynamics of "selective inattention" that perpetuate gaps in awareness and dissociative states of self (Bromberg, 2011). Donnell Stern describes "unformulated" realms of experience that operate out of awareness, never having been articulated or integrated into the conscious sense of self (2015). Drawing on empirical lines of study in the fields of neuroscience, thinkers increasingly encompass the dynamics of interoception, emotion, and non-verbal modes of communication in formulations of implicit processes.

Over the years, relational thinkers have reformulated conceptions of defense, emphasizing the dynamics of anxiety, behavior, and interpersonal life. Adler had described "safeguarding tendencies" that regulate the experience of vulnerability and inferiority in developing his social perspective. Winnicott thought of the "false self" as a defensive mode of adaptation. Sullivan centered on protective restrictions of consciousness in the organization of the "self-system" and in his formulations of "selective inattention." Interpersonal thinkers have continued to expand conceptions of dissociation and multiple self states. Object relations theorists, influenced by Klein and Fairbairn, have emphasized the defensive functions of splitting and projective identification.

Although a range of perspectives have shaped formulations of defense across the schools of thought, practitioners emphasize that any feelings, thoughts, or actions that shift attention from threatening experience can serve defensive functions. As Jonathan Shedler observes, "There is nothing at all mysterious about defensive processes. Defense is as simple as not noticing something, not thinking about something, not putting two and two together, or simply distracting ourselves with something else" (2006, p. 28).

Converging lines of study across the fields of neuroscience, developmental psychology, cognitive psychology, social psychology, and experimental psychology corroborate core propositions underlying conceptions of personality that shape understanding in the relational paradigm, emphasizing the fundamental role of attachment in the emergence of the self; mental representations of self, others, and modes of interactive experience; the origins of basic dispositions in childhood; and the ways in which unconscious motivations, emotions, and thoughts influence the dynamics of defensive processes and patterns of behavior (for reviews of empirical research see Curtis, 2020; Fonagy & Target, 2007; Fonagy, Roth & Higgitt, 2005; Luborsky & Barett, 2006; Schore, 2019a,

2019b; Shedler, 2010; Solms, 2018a, 2018b; Weinberg & Westen, 2001; Westen, 1998, 2005).

Health, Well-Being, and Optimal Functioning

Clinical scholars encompass subjective states of experience, inner representations of self and others, and patterns of interpersonal behavior in conceptions of health, well-being, and optimal functioning. Thinkers focus on the development of core structures of personality and corresponding capacities for relationship believed to influence patterns of feeling, thinking, and acting. The fully functioning person is characterized by a cohesive sense of self and identity; the capacity to regulate emotion and express the range of feeling; affirming but realistic views and expectations of self and others; stable patterns of interpersonal behavior, and fulfilling relationships. Flexible ways of being and relating facilitate efforts to form attachments, participate in social life, assimilate new experiences, and pursue meaningful goals. Some thinkers emphasize concepts of "effectance," focusing on the development of capacities for mastery and self-efficacy (Curtis, 2020; Greenberg, 1991). As we have seen, Winnicott and Kohut encompass the realms of subjectivity in their accounts of health and well-being, focusing on the experience of cohesion, coherence, and continuity in states of self; embodiment and the sense of aliveness; capacities for agency, initiative, creativity, and play; and the ability to generate ways of being that we register as authentic and meaningful, originating deeply within us.

More broadly, relational thinkers recognize the sustaining functions of relationship and community across the course of life. Like Adler and Ferenczi, many of the early psychoanalysts were progressive activists, deeply engaged in social and cultural concerns. Horney, Sullivan and Fromm bridged psychological and social domains of concern in shaping their versions of interpersonal psychoanalysis, linking the health and well-being of the individual with values and patterns of life in community and culture. Paul Wachtel, continuing lines of social criticism established in the interpersonal school, has explored the dynamics of racism, class, individualism, and consumerism in American society over the last three decades. In doing so he has challenged scholars and clinicians to expand conceptions of health, well-being, and the common good, taking more account of the ways in which social, political, cultural, and economic conditions influence the course of development, health, vulnerability, and problems in living (Wachel, 1989, 1999, 2014; see Altman, 2009; Borden, 2009; Danto, 2005; and Safran, 2012, for expanded discussion of social criticism and activism in the psychoanalytic tradition).

Vulnerability, Psychopathology, and Problems in Living

Thinkers distinguish predisposing, precipitating, and perpetuating conditions in formulating conceptions of vulnerability and psychopathology. In accord with Freud's notion of "overdetermination," clinicians realize that problems in living are influenced by a range of factors, including constitution and temperament; the dynamics of attachment, relational life, social surrounds, and culture; traumatic events; restrictions of opportunity; and current stressors. In line with Freud's formulation of "multiple function," therapists assume that particular patterns of behavior potentially carry different meanings and serve a range of purposes. A recurring symptom, for example, may preserve coherence and continuity in sense of self, regulate fear and anxiety, reduce feelings of hopelessness and helplessness, and restore self-esteem (see McWilliams, 2004, 2020, on psychoanalytic conceptions of assessment, diagnosis, and case formulation).

Developmental perspectives continue to shape conceptions of vulnerability and problems in living across the different schools of thought. Some thinkers, drawing on the formulations of Winnicott and Kohut, emphasize "arrests" or "deficits" in the development of the self that compromise ways of being and relating. As we have seen, Winnicott centers on the ways in which cumulative trauma undermines the emergence of the self, and he distinguishes "true self" and "false self" states of experience in his formulations of authenticity, defensive processes, and psychopathology. Kohut links structural deficits in the organization of the self to earlier lapses in care that limit the development of capacities to regulate emotion, generate meaning, and engage in relational life.

Object relations theorists center on internalized representations of interpersonal experience and defensive processes, such as splitting and projective identification, thought to perpetuate problems in living. Fairbairn proposes that basic modes of connection, established in the past, are structured as representations of self and others, guiding perceptions of others and patterns of behavior. He describes "splits" in the representational world of relational life that compromise the integrity of the self. The individual interprets situations along the lines of earlier relationships, and the ongoing cycle of projection and re-internalization of self-other configurations shapes the course of relational life. Bowlby emphasizes the ways in which rigid working models of self, other, and modes of interactive experience distort perceptions of others and constrict ways of being, relating, and living.

Interpersonal thinkers center on outer domains of experience, attending to the dynamics of anxiety, dissociation, and particular patterns of "me-you" behavior that precipitate maladaptive patterns of feeling, thought, and action. Wachtel, drawing on Sullivan's formulations, emphasizes the role of fear and defensive operations that lead to avoidance of experience, compromising the development of crucial skills in living. Sullivan was critical of the disease model inherited from medicine, preferring the phrase "problems in living" over diagnostic classifications of mental disorders. As noted, he speaks of "dynamisms of difficulty;" Horney and Wachtel describe "vicious circles" of behavior. They think of dysfunction as a dynamic, cyclical process in which "feared and anticipated relational events tend to be elicited and enacted" in interaction with others, who respond in complementary ways (Messer & Warren, 1995, p. 119–120). Ironically, patterns of interaction perpetuate negative perceptions of experience and reinforce maladaptive behavior. Sullivan and Wachtel empha-size the role of learning in development, change, and growth, converging with orienting perspectives in the behavioral paradigm, emphasizing the development of capacities and skills through in-vivo experience.

As we have seen, the relational field is the fundamental organizer of per-sonality and self, and researchers have documented the ways in which the dynamics of attachment, interactive experience, and social surrounds shape the course of development. The first generation of relational thinkers focused largely on critical periods of care in infancy and early childhood in formulat-ing their understanding of vulnerability and problems in functioning. Over the years, however, following critiques of theory and research, investigators have broadened the scope of study to consider the ways in which relation-ships, life events, trauma, and social conditions influence the dynamics of development and problems in living across the course of life (Borden, 2009; Curtis, 2020).

Although researchers continue to explore the adverse effects of deprivation and trauma, relational thinkers have increasingly recognized the organizing and sustaining functions of maladaptive behavior. Following Mitchell's for-mulations, clinicians assume that psychopathology is self-perpetuating because it is embedded in global ways of being, relating, and living elaborated over the course of development. He emphasizes the "pervasive tendency to preserve the continuity, connections, and familiarity of one's personal, interactional world" (Mitchell, 1988, p. 33; see Borden, 2009, for case studies).

However limiting "vicious circles" of thought, feeling, and behavior may be, Mitchell proposes that established ways of being and relating serve crucial functions, helping us to preserve cohesion and continuity in sense of self and subjective experience; maintain connections with internalized representations of others, and provide safety and security as we negotiate the dynamics of interpersonal life. From the perspective of object relations theory, we perpe-tuate particular patterns of behavior in efforts to preserve connections with internal representations and presences of others. "What is new is frightening because it requires what one experiences as the abandonment of old loyalties, through which one feels connected and devoted" (Mitchell, 1988, p. 291). In the domain of interpersonal life, we perpetuate particular patterns of interaction in efforts to regulate fear and anxiety and maximize safety and security. Following Sullivan's formulation, "security operations steer (the individual) into familiar channels and away from the anxiety-shrouded unknown" (Mitchell, 1988, p. 291; see Borden, 2009, for expanded discus-sion and case studies).

Therapeutic Action

Although psychodynamically oriented practitioners focus on circumscribed symptoms, concerns, and problems in living, the therapeutic process carries the potential to foster the development of capacities and skills instrumental in ongoing growth and individuation of the self. Clinicians assume that the core conditions and activities of psychodynamic therapy: 1) deepen awareness of unconscious realms of experience, encompassing motivations, sensations, feelings, thoughts, imagery, and behavior that perpetuate problems in functioning; 2) strengthen capacities to register, process, and regulate subjective experience; 3) reorganize unconscious associational networks that underlie structures of meaning, including motives, schemas, and models of self, others, and interactive experience; 4) engage inner and outer realms of experience that precipitate fear and anxiety, restricting ranges of behavior and opportunity; 5) expand coping capacities and problem-solving skills; and 6) strengthen relational capacities, patterns of interpersonal functioning, and social networks.

The relational schools of thought encompass orienting perspectives and fundamental concerns that have shaped psychoanalytic understanding from the beginning, and we rediscover points of connection with the contributions of Freud and Jung as we review formulations of therapeutic action across the broader paradigm.

Concepts of therapeutic action, change, and growth emphasize the role of the relationship and the dynamics of interactive experience; use of associative methods that foster processing of subjective experience, exploration of implicit memory, and the development of emotional insight; and various forms of activity and experiential learning that strengthen capacities and skills instrumental in problem-solving, coping, and growth.

The Therapeutic Relationship and the Dynamics of Interactive Experience

Clinical scholars emphasize the multiple functions of the therapeutic relationship and the dynamics of interactive experience in efforts to negotiate problems in living, strengthen capacities and skills, and work toward change and growth. The therapeutic relationship facilitates growth in a variety of ways, providing crucial sources of experience, learning, and understanding. Practitioners emphasize the critical functions of the therapeutic alliance and the constancy of care in the holding environment; the role of experiential learning through interpersonal interaction; and open-ended dialogue and co-creation of meaning that deepens understanding of self, interpersonal behavior, and life experience (see Norcross & Wampold, 2018).The concept of the therapeutic alliance originates in the psychodynamic tradition, as noted in Chapter 1. Researchers encompassed three domains of concern in their formulations of the alliance: the attachment bond between the patient and the therapist; mutual agreement on the goals of treatment; and shared understanding of the rationale and core activities of the therapeutic process (Horvath, 2006). Following the emergence of the relational paradigm, however, practitioners have come to think of the therapeutic alliance as an ongoing *process* of reflection and negotiation between the patient and therapist about the goals and activities of treatment, recognizing the mutuality of the relationship and the collaborative nature of the therapeutic process (Borden, 2009; Safran, 2012).

From the perspective of self psychology, the practitioner's empathic attunement and responsiveness as a "selfobject" strengthen the cohesion and integrity of the self and the development of capacities to regulate emotion. The experience of presence, empathic attunement, and synchrony in therapeutic interaction and the constancy of care in the holding environment are thought to strengthen capacities to regulate sensation and emotion, emphasized in accounts of nonverbal, interactive forms of communication mediated by the right hemisphere of the brain (Schore, 2019b). In line with research on the dynamics of attachment and caregiving in infancy, the therapist and patient provide mutual regulation through reciprocal patterns of interaction and communication.

From the perspective of object relations psychology, the practitioner and patient co-create reparative experiences over the course of interaction that modify inner models of self and others, reorganize dysfunctional patterns of defense, and foster more functional ways of being, relating, and living. New and different ways of relating are thought to alter the associative pathways of neural networks that mediate subjective states, representations of self and others, and defensive processes.

From the perspective of the interpersonal school, the practitioner is inevitably engaged in the patient's representative patterns of behavior in the relational field of the therapeutic process. Following Sullivan's formulations, we think of the clinician as a participant-observer, and emphasize the reciprocal nature of therapeutic interaction. Ongoing interaction between the patient and therapist facilitates efforts to identify "vicious circles" of behavior and strengthen capacities to process experience, regulate emotion, and negotiate interpersonal life. The therapist encourages the patient to "try something different," to explore new interpersonal situations where richer experiences of self and others are possible (Mitchell, 1988, p. 290).

Formulations of transference and countertransference states in object relations thought and interpersonal psychoanalysis center on inner models of relational life and the reciprocal nature of interactive experience in the social field. From the perspective of object relations theory, conceptions of transference emphasize the ways in which inner models of self and others influence perceptions of experience, constructions of meaning, and patterns of interpersonal behavior. From the perspective of the interpersonal school, formulations of transference emphasize patterns of learning and expectation established over the course of relational life. As noted earlier, research in the field of cognitive neuroscience provides empirical support for the foregoing formulations of transference. To the degree that the therapeutic relationship corresponds to prototypes of earlier relational life, it is likely to activate similar patterns of motivation, emotion, thought, conflict, defense, and interpersonal behavior (Luborsky & Barrett, 2006; Shedler, 2010; Solms, 2018a; Westen, 2005; Westen & Gabbard, 2002a, 2002b).

Clinicians conceptualize countertransference states as role-responsive complements or counterparts to the patient's ways of being and relating, generating experience that deepens understanding of inner life and interactive processes perpetuating dysfunctional patterns of thought, feeling, and action. Enactments of behavior in the therapeutic process, originating in intrapsychic conflict, earlier relationships, restrictions of opportunity, or trauma, facilitate efforts to clarify maladaptive modes of interaction and to strengthen capacities and skills in negotiating interpersonal life. In contrast to notions of neutrality that had shaped classical models of therapeutic action, contemporary relational thinkers assume that clinicians inevitably join patients in enactments, realizing the influence of complex, nonverbal, implicit patterns of communication that operate out of awareness.

Over the course of the therapeutic process, researchers propose, the patient internalizes positive elements of the therapeutic relationship, modifying inner representations of self and others, and develops capacities and skills through experiential learning that strengthen efforts to manage vulnerability and negotiate problems in living. From the perspective of neuroscience, as noted, the core activities of the therapeutic process are thought to alter the structure and function of associative networks established over the course of development, facilitating the reorganization and integration of neural pathways instrumental in emotional regulation and functional behavior. The intrapsychic domain of the relational matrix is transformed as the patient relinquishes ties to past forms of relation.

From the beginnings of psychotherapy, psychoanalytically oriented practitioners have recognized the fundamental importance of unstructured dialogue, narrative, and the creation of meaning in change and growth. Freud thought of the patient as a narrator and the therapist as a co-author, describing his ways of working as a literary method. Relational perspectives emphasize the ways in which the therapist and patient render experience into words and co-create narrative accounts of events through the ongoing construction and elaboration of stories. The aim of the process is to help patients reformulate life experience in ways that strengthen the sense of personal agency and deepen understanding of the origins, meanings, and implications of current concerns, and "to do so in a way that makes change conceivable and attainable" (Schafer, 1980, p. 38). What is crucial is not the "historical truthfulness" of the account but rather the "narrative coherence" and adaptive functions of the story (see Borden, 1999, 2000, 2009, 2010; Coles, 1997; Spence, 1982).

Following efforts to bridge psychodynamic and behavioral perspectives in integrative models of practice, clinicians have come to think of observational learning, modeling, and reinforcement as formative processes in the patient-therapist interaction. The working alliance serves as a catalyst, helping the patient more fully engage the core activities of the therapeutic process. As we will see shortly, practitioners increasingly emphasize use of tasks outside of sessions to facilitate development of crucial skills in living (Borden, 2009, 2014; Wachtel, 2011, 2014).

In line with conceptions of therapeutic action proposed by Jung and Ferenczi, relational thinkers realize the ways in which the patient and the practitioner shape the process and outcomes of help and care, and conceptions of the relationship acknowledge mutual sources of recognition, empathy, and influence. In doing so, they deepen appreciation of intersubjectivity and mutuality in the therapeutic process. The focus on the dynamics of the therapeutic relationship and current patterns of interaction distinguish contemporary relational models of intervention from classical Freudian approaches that emphasize principles of neutrality and interpretation of transference and resistance in accord with the propositions of drive psychology.

Clinical scholars have increasingly recognized the personal characteristics and immediate emotional experience of the therapist. As Jon Mills observes in his account of relational psychoanalysis, practitioners emphasize "a natural, humane, and authentic" manner of engagement in the therapeutic process, finding therapists "more revelatory, interactive, and inclined to disclose accounts of their own experience, ... enlist and solicit perceptions from the patient about their own subjective comportment, and generally acknowledge how a patient's responsiveness and demeanor is triggered by the purported attitudes, sensibility, and behavior" of the therapist (Mills, 2005, p. 155). The clinician's ongoing exploration of enactments, transference and countertransference states, and the patient's experience of the clinician has expanded conceptions of the therapeutic process.

Free Association

Methods of free association allow the therapist and patient to explore the dynamics of unconscious processes that perpetuate particular ways of feeling, thinking, and acting. Drawing on techniques that Freud introduced in his formulations of therapeutic practice, clinicians use free association in efforts to process implicit realms of experience, advising patients to speak freely about whatever comes to mind, even if it does not seem to make sense, without judgment, much as we would instruct in mindfulness meditation. The goal is to help patients recognize and challenge defenses and resistance, bringing unconscious experience more fully into awareness, rendering implicit experience into words.

The clinician and patient process elements from the flow of associations, enactments, transference and countertransference states, and varying forms of resistance, bringing new meaning to experience. In formulating unconscious realms of experience, we assume, patients reorganize associative connections across neural networks and deepen awareness of motives, feelings, thoughts, dreams, fantasies, and goals that expand understanding of self, relational life, past experience, and anticipated future. Carefully focused questions, observations, and formulations convey the clinician's efforts to understand the potential meanings carried in manifest content of words and actions operating out of awareness, deepening insight and understanding. Some practitioners have modified classical methods of free association in briefer forms of psychotherapy, selecting particular feelings, thoughts, or memories for associative exploration (Westen, 2005).

Although classical Freudian conceptions of therapeutic action continue to emphasize the curative functions of interpretation, relational thinkers have increasingly recognized the critical role of the therapeutic relationship, colla-boration, and interactive experience in the mutual creation of meaning and understanding, focusing on the functional outcomes of formulations and nar-ratives. In line with the constructivist perspectives that had shaped postmodern thought at the end of the 20th century, therapists have come to think of interpretations as co-created constructions of meaning rather than as author-itative accounts of underlying truths or realities. The patient and clinician collaborate in their efforts to make sense of experience, working to deepen awareness and understanding.

Practitioners make a distinction between cognitive insight and emotional insight, emphasizing the experiential features of the therapeutic process. Reviews of research comparing the outcomes of traditional cognitive-beha-vioral treatment and psychodynamic psychotherapy suggest that the beneficial effects of cognitive insight tend to diminish over time, whereas emotional insight, linking the domains of thought and feeling, is more likely to bring about enduring change and ongoing growth (Shedler, 2010, 2015; Solms, 2018a, 2018b). As noted in Chapter 3, the capacity to experience emotion and to tolerate "optimal stress" is thought to enhance neuroplasticity across the course of life.

Activity and Experiential Learning

Freud and Jung were more active in their ways of working than many clinicians realize, and the first generation of psychoanalytic thinkers recognized the cri-tical importance of experiential learning and problem-solving in their concep-tions of change and growth. As we have seen, Adler, Rank, and Ferenczi introduced active methods of intervention over the course of their practice. Psychodynamically oriented clinicians have increasingly drawn on cognitive and behavioral approaches in efforts to expand concepts of therapeutic action and help patients generate activity in everyday life. Practitioners may challenge dysfunctional beliefs and fears that perpetuate avoidance of experiential opportunities, engage in mutual problem-solving, or propose activities that foster the development of capacities and skills. Clinicians increasingly empha-size the crucial role of activity in efforts to deepen insight and strengthen the development of capacities and skills (Wachtel, 2014; see review of behavioral concepts of therapeutic action in Chapter 6, this volume). As Wachtel observes: "Overt behavior and intrapsychic processes are not really separate realms. They are most fully understood in relation to each other and in terms of the complex feedback loops that link and maintain them" (2011, p. 338).

Neuroscience and Therapeutic Action

As we have seen, psychodynamically oriented practitioners emphasize the cru-cial functions of the therapeutic relationship, interactive experience, and the constancy of care in the holding environment. Presumably, the empathic attunement and synchrony of the therapeutic relationship activate bonding processes that mediate the dynamics of attachment and carry the potential to reinstate neural growth, helping patients strengthen capacities to process and integrate subjective experience, regulate emotion, and negotiate relational life. Following developments in attachment research described in Chapters 2 and 3, practitioners increasingly consider the role of unconscious, non-verbal, right brain functions in their conceptions of the therapeutic alliance, intersubjectivity, communication, and change.

In accord with the proposal that moderate arousal or "optimal stress" enhances the properties of neuroplasticity, clinicians emphasize the role of emotion in conceptions of therapeutic action, change and growth, distinguishing "cognitive insight" from "emotional insight." As discussed earlier, practitioners intensify emotion as they explore the dynamics of defense, process interactive experience, and offer formulations and interpretations of behavior. Thinkers describe various forms of challenge that carry implicit or explicit suggestions for change. Clinicians may explore beliefs and assumptions that fail to take account of actual circumstances, for example, or focus on feelings, thoughts, and experiences that perpetuate problems in living.

Some psychodynamically oriented clinicians integrate cognitive and behavioral methods in efforts to help patients engage aspects of inner life or outer experience they have avoided out of fear, as discussed earlier. In doing so practitioners encourage the patient to register, recognize, and express a wider range of feelings, creating conditions of mild to moderate stress thought to activate the production of neurotransmitters and neural growth hormones associated with long-term potentiation, learning, and cortical reorganization.

Psychodynamic approaches engage interoceptive, emotional, cognitive, and behavioral processes thought to be instrumental in "top-down" and "bottom-up" modes of integration, reorganizing the structures of associational networks established over the course of development, fostering the formation of new, adaptive linkages and patterns of behavior (Cozolino, 2017; Schore, 2019a, 2019b; Westen, 2005; Westen & Gabbard, 2002a, 2002b). The patient and clinician process experience in accord with Freud's classic account of therapeutic action, "Remembering, repeating, and working through" (1914/1958), exploring the discontinuities and dissociations of unconscious and conscious processes through free association and interpretation, integrating and reorganizing neural networks that mediate the dynamics of motivation, emotion, thought, defense, and behavior.

From the perspective of cognitive neuroscience, therapeutic action challenges connections between mental processes that have become linked through experience over time, perpetuating problems in functioning. The core activities of the "working through" process are thought to weaken links between nodes of association that have been structured over the course of experience, lowering their levels of activation, fostering the development of new associative connections that strengthen underdeveloped links across neural structures instrumental in change and growth. Structural change does not replace earlier networks; rather, the reorganization of networks deactivates problematic links and activates new, adaptive connections (see Gabbard & Westen, 2003, pp. 827–829).

From a narrative perspective, as we have seen, the therapist and the patient collaborate in ongoing efforts to process experience, construct meaning, and elaborate life stories that foster change and growth. As noted, researchers propose that the dynamics of narrative engage the functions of the right and left hemispheres, fostering the integration of neural networks throughout the brain. The autonoetic, analogical, mentalizing functions of the right hemisphere shape the imagery and themes of narratives, while the left hemisphere mediates interpretive and linguistic processing of content (Siegel, 2020).

Beyond the experiential opportunities of the therapeutic process, as we have seen, thinkers have increasingly realized the ways in which the relationships, activities, and practices of everyday life carry the potential to strengthen the development of capacities and skills, fostering neural integration, insight, and growth. Integrative conceptions of psychodynamic therapy increasingly combine cognitive and behavioral methods in efforts to generate new forms of action, experience, and learning in the outer world. As in the other foundational schools of thought, integrative approaches potentially include a range of "bottom-up" practices believed to engage subcortical regions of sensation and emotion, including use of the breath, mindfulness meditation, yoga, walking, and artistic and musical activities.

Concluding Comments

Over the last three decades, as we have seen, reformulations of psychodynamic thought have brought about major shifts in theoretical formulations, research, and practice. Clinical scholars have increasingly focused on conceptions of mind, self, relationship, and social life in their reformulations of theory, emphasizing the dynamics of unconscious emotional and cognitive processes and the crucial role of attachment and experiential learning across the course of development.

Pragmatic sensibilities shaped our earliest methods of therapeutic practice, and contemporary approaches converge with essential concerns in the formulations of clinical pragmatism I have described here. Clinicians challenge reductive formulations of help and care based on a technical rationalism and standardized models of intervention in reductive versions of evidence-based practice, drawing on comparative approaches to understanding. Concepts of therapeutic action focus on the subjectivity and agency of the individual; the crucial role of the relationship, collaboration, open-ended dialogue, and interactive experience; co-creation of narrative and meaning; and various kinds of experiential learning instrumental in the development of capacities, skills, and realization of potential. Practitioners continue to integrate ideas and methods from cognitive, behavioral, and humanistic schools of thought in efforts to strengthen the outcomes of help and care.

References

Adler, A. (1927/1992). *Understanding human nature* (C. Brett, Trans.). Oxford: Oneworld Publications.

Altman, N. (2009). *The analyst in the inner city*, 2nd edn. New York: Routledge.

Aron, L. & Harris, A. (2011a). *Relational psychoanalysis IV: Expansion of theory*. Hove: Psychology Press.

Aron, L. & Harris, A. (2011b). *Relational psychoanalysis V: Evolution of process*. Hove: Psychology Press.

Aron, L. & Lechich, M. (2012). Relational psychoanalysis, in G. Gabbard, B. Litowitz & P. Williams (Eds.), *Textbook of psychoanalysis* (pp. 211–224). Washington, DC: American Psychiatric Publishing.

Barness, R. (Ed.) (2018). *Core competencies of relational psychoanalysis*. New York: Routledge.

Beebe, B. & Lachman, M. (2013). *Infant research and adult treatment: Co-constructing interactions*. New York: Routledge.

Belkin, M. & White, C. (Eds.) (2020) *Intersectionality and relational psychoanalysis: New perspectives on race, gender and sexuality*. New York: Routledge.

Benjamin, L. (1993). *Diagnosis and treatment of personality disorders: A structural approach*. New York: Guilford.

Blatt, S. & Homan, E. (1992). Parent-child interactions in the etiology of dependent and self-critical depression. *Clinical Psychology Review*, 12, 47–91.

Bollas, C. (1989). *Forces of destiny*. London: Free Association Books.

Borden, W. (1999). Pluralism, pragmatism, and the therapeutic endeavor in brief dynamic treatment, in W. Borden (Ed.), *Comparative approaches in brief dynamic psychotherapy* (pp. 7–42). New York: Haworth.

Borden, W. (2000). The relational paradigm in contemporary psychoanalysis: Toward a psychodynamically-informed social work perspective. *Social Service Review*, 74 (3), 352–379.

Borden, W. (2009). *Contemporary psychodynamic theory and practice: Toward a critical pluralism*. New York: Oxford University Press.

Borden, W. (2010). Taking multiplicity seriously: Pluralism, pragmatism, and integrative perspectives in social work practice, in W. Borden (Ed). *Reshaping theory in contemporary social work* (pp. 3–25). New York: Columbia University Press.

Borden, W. (2018). The Independent Tradition in British psychoanalysis: Therapeutic action and clinical pragmatism. Lecture, Fellows Program in Advanced Psychodynamic Psychotherapy, Chicago, IL, University of Chicago.

Borden, W. & Clark, J. (2012). Contemporary psychodynamic theory, research, and practice, in T. Rzepnicki, S. McCracken, & H. Briggs (Eds.), *From task-centered social work to evidence-based and integrative practice* (pp. 65–88). New York: Oxford University Press.

Bowlby, J. (1988). *A secure base*. New York: Basic Books.

Bromberg, P. (2011). *The shadow of the tsunami: And the growth of the relational mind*. New York: Routledge.

Coles, R. (1997). *Doing documentary work*. New York: Oxford University Press.

Cozolino, L. (2017). *The neuroscience of psychotherapy*, 3rd edn. New York: Norton.

Curtis, R. (2020). Relational psychanalytic/psychodynamic psychotherapy, in S. Messer & N. Kaslow (Eds). *Essential psychotherapies* (pp. 71–108). New York: Guilford.

Danto, E. (2005). *Freud's free clinics*. New York: Columbia University Press.

Fairbairn, W. R. D. (1952). A synopsis of the development of the author's views regarding the structure of the personality, in W. R. D. Fairbairn, *Psychoanalytic studies of the personality* (pp. 162–182). London: Tavistock.

Ferenczi, S. (1932/1949). The confusion of tongues between adults and the child: The language of tenderness and passion, *International Journal of Psycho-Analysis*, 30 (4), 225–230.

Fonagy, P. (2001). *Attachment theory and psychoanalysis.* New York: Other Press.

Fonagy, P. & Target, M. (2007). The rooting of the mind in the body: New links between attachment theory and psychoanalytic thought. *Journal of the American Psychoanalytic Association*, 55 (2), 411–456.

Freud, S. (1914/1958). Remembering, repeating, and working through, in J. Strachey (Ed. & Trans.), *The standard edition of the complete psychological works of Sigmund Freud*, Vol. 12 (pp. 145–157). London: Hogarth Press.

Gabbard, G. & Westen, D. (2003). Rethinking therapeutic action. *International Journal of Psychoanalysis*, 84, 823–841.

Gibbons, M., Crits-Christoph, P. & Hearon, B. (2008). The empirical status of psychodynamic therapies. *Annual Review of Clinical Psychology*, 4, 93–108.

Greenberg, J. (1991). *Oedipus and beyond.* Cambridge, MA: Harvard University Press.

Greenberg, J. & Mitchell, S. (1983). *Object relations in psychoanalysis.* Cambridge, MA: Harvard University Press.

Harris, A. (2011). The relational turn: Landscape and cannon. *Journal of the American Psychoanalytic Association*, 4, 701–736.

Horney, K. (1950). *Neurosis and human growth.* New York: Norton.

Horvath, A. (2006). The alliance in context: Accomplishments, challenges, and future directions. *Psychotherapy theory, research, practice, training*, 43 (3), 258–263.

Kohut, H. (1971). *The analysis of self.* New York: International Universities Press.

Kohut, H. (1977). *The restoration of the self.* Madison, CT: International Universities Press.

Kohut, H. (1984). *How does analysis cure?* Chicago, IL: University of Chicago Press.

Leichsenring, F. (2009). Psychodynamic psychotherapy: A review of efficacy and effectiveness studies, in R. A. Levy & S. J. Ablon (Eds.), *Handbook of evidence-based psychodynamic therapy* (pp. 3–27). New York: Humana Press.

Leichsenring, F. & Rabung, S. (2009). Effectiveness of long-term psychodynamic psychotherapy: A meta-analysis. *Journal of the American Medical Association*, 300 (13), 1587–1589.

Levenson, H. (2017). *Brief dynamic therapy*, 2nd edn. Washington, DC: American Psychological Association.

Luborsky, L. & Barrett, M. (2006). The history and empirical status of key psychoanalytic concepts, *Annual Review of Clinical Psychology*, 2, 1–19.

Luborsky, L. & Crits-Christoph, P. (1990). *Understanding transference: The CCRT method.* New York: Basic Books.

Masling, J. & Bornstein, R. (1994). *Empirical perspectives on object relations theory.* Washington, DC: American Psychological Association.

McWilliams, N. (2004). *Psychoanalytic psychotherapy.* New York: Guilford.

McWilliams, N. (2020). *Psychiatric diagnosis*, 2nd edn. New York: Guilford.

Messer, S. & Kaslow, N. (2020). Current issues in psychotherapy: Theory, research, and practice, in S. Messer & N. Kaslow (Eds.), *Essential psychotherapies* (pp. 3–32). New York: Guilford.

Messer, S. & Warren, S. (1995). *Models of brief psychodynamic psychotherapy.* New York: Guilford.

Mills, J. (2005). A critique of relational psychoanalysis. *Psychoanalytic Psychology*, 22 (2), 155–188.

Mitchell, S. (1988). *Relational concepts in psychoanalysis.* Cambridge, MA: Harvard University Press.

Mitchell, S. (1991). Editorial philosophy. *Psychoanalytic Dialogues*, 1, 1–7.

Mitchell, S. (1993). *Hope and dread in psychoanalysis.* New York: Basic Books.

Mitchell, S. (1997). *Influence and autonomy in psychoanalysis.* Hillsdale, NJ: Analytic Press.

Mitchell, S. (2000). *Relationality.* Hillsdale, NJ: Analytic Press.

Mitchell, S. & Aron, L. (1999). *Relational psychoanalysis: The emergence of a tradition.* Hillsdale, NJ: Analytic Press.

Mitchell, S. & Harris, A. (2004). What's American about American psychoanalysis? *Psychoanalytic Dialogues*, 14, 165–191.

Norcross, J. & Wampold, B. (2018). A new therapy for each patient: Evidence based relationships and responsiveness. *Journal of Clinical Psychology*, 74, 1889–1906.

Rank, O. (1936). *Will therapy* (J. Taft, Trans.). New York: Knopf.

Roth, A. & Fonagy, P. (2005). *What works for whom? A critical review of psychotherapy research*, 2nd edn. New York: Guilford Press.

Safran, J. (2012). *Psychoanalysis and psychoanalytic therapies.* Washington, DC: American Psychological Association.

Schafer, R. (1980). Narration in the psychoanalytic dialogue. *Critical Inquiry*, 7, 29–53.

Schore, A. (2003a). *Affect dysregulation and disorders of the self.* New York: Norton.

Schore, A. (2003b). *Affect regulation and the repair of the self.* New York: Norton.

Schore, A. (2012). *The science of the art of psychotherapy.* New York: Norton.

Schore, A. (2019a). *The development of the unconscious mind.* New York: Norton.

Schore, A. (2019b). *Right brain psychotherapy.* New York: Norton.

Shedler, J. (2006). *That was then, this is now: An introduction to contemporary psychodynamic psychotherapy for the rest of us.* Retrieved from //jonathanshedler.com/writings/ (accessed March 3, 2019).

Shedler, J. (2010). The efficacy of psychodynamic psychotherapy. *American Psychologist* 65 (2), 98–109.

Shedler, J. (2015). Where is the evidence for evidence-based therapy? *Journal of Psychological Therapies in Primary Care*, 4, 47–59.

Siegel, D. (2020). *The developing mind*, 3rd edn. New York: Guilford.

Solms, M. (2018a) The scientific standing of psychoanalysis. *British Journal of Psychiatry International*, 15, 5–8.

Solms, M. (2018b). The neurobiological underpinnings of psychoanalytic theory and therapy. *Frontiers in Behavioral Neuroscience*, 12, 294.

Spence, D. (1982). *Narrative truth and historical truth.* New York: Norton.

Sroufe, A. (2016). The place of attachment in development, in J. Cassidy & P. R. Shaver (Eds.), *Handbook of attachment: Theory, research, and clinical applications*, 3rd edn (pp. 997–1011). New York: Guilford.

Sroufe, A., Egelund, B., Carlson, E. & Collins, A. (2005). *The development of the person.* New York: Guilford.

Stern, D. B. (2015). *Relational freedom: Emerging properties of the interpersonal field.* New York: Routledge.

Stern, D. N. (1985). *The interpersonal world of the infant.* New York: Basic.

Stern, D. N. (2004). *The present moment in psychotherapy and everyday life.* New York: Norton.

Stolorow & Atwood (1992). *Contexts of being: The intersubjective foundations of psychological life.* Hillside, NJ: Analytic Press.

Strupp, H. & Binder, J. (1984). *Psychotherapy in a new key.* New York: Basic Books.

Sullivan, H. S. (1953). *The interpersonal theory of psychiatry.* New York: Norton.

Suttie, I. (1935). *The origins of love and hate.* London: Kegan Paul.

Wachtel, P. (1989). *The poverty of affluence.* Philadelphia, PA: New Society Publishers.

Wachtel, P. (1999). *Race in the mind of America.* New York: Routledge.

Wachtel, P. (2008). *Relational theory and the practice of psychotherapy.* New York: Guilford.

Wachtel, P. (2011). *Therapeutic communication*, 2nd edn. New York: Guilford.

Wachtel, P. (2014). *Cyclical psychodynamics and the contextual self.* New York: Routledge.

Wampold, B. (2015). How important are the common factors in psychotherapy? An update. *World Psychiatry*, 14 (3), 270–277.

Weinberg, J. & Westen, D. (2001). Science and psychodynamics: From arguments about Freud to data. *Psychological Inquiry*, 12 (3), 129–132.

Westen, D. (1998). The scientific legacy of Sigmund Freud: Toward a psychodynamically-informed psychological science. *Psychological Bulletin*, 124 (3), 333–371.

Westen, D. (2005). Implications of research in cognitive neuroscience for psychodynamic psychology, in G. Gabbard, J. Beck & J. Holmes (Eds.), *Oxford textbook of psychotherapy* (pp. 443–448). New York: Oxford University Press.

Westen, D. (2007). Discovering what works in the community: Toward a general partnership of clinicians and researchers, in S. G Hofmann & J. Weinberger (Eds.), *The art and science of psychotherapy* (pp. 3–30). New York: Routledge.

Westen, D. & Bradley, R. (2005). Empirically-supported complexity: Rethinking evidence-based practice in psychotherapy. *Current Directions in Psychological Science*, 14 (5), 266–271.

Westen, D. & Gabbard, G. (2002a). Developments in cognitive neuroscience: Conflict, compromise, and connectionism. *Journal of the American Psychoanalytic Association*, 50, 53–90.

Westen, D. & Gabbard, G. (2002b). Developments in cognitive neuroscience: Implications for theories of transference. *Journal of the American Psychoanalytic Association*, 50, 99–134.

Westen, D., Novotny, C. M. & Thompson-Brenner, H. (2004). The empirical status of empirically supported psychotherapies: Assumptions, findings, and reporting in controlled clinical trials. *Psychological Bulletin*, 130 (4), 631–663.

Winnicott, D. W. (1945/1975). Primitive emotional development, in D. W. Winnicott, *Through pediatrics to psychoanalysis* (pp. 145–156). New York: Basic.

Winnicott, D. W. (1952/1975). Anxiety associated with insecurity, in D. W. Winnicott, *Through paediatrics to psychoanalysis* (pp. 97–100). New York: Basic.

Winnicott, D. W. (1963/1965). A theory of psychiatric disorder, in D. W. Winnicott, *The maturational process and the facilitating environment* (pp. 230–242). New York: International Universities Press.

Winnicott, D. W. (1971). *Therapeutic consultations in child psychiatry.* New York: Basic Books.

Wolitzky, D. & Eagle, M. (1997). Psychoanalytic theories of psychotherapy, in P. Wachtel & S. Messer (Eds.), *Theories of psychotherapy* (pp. 39–96). Washington, DC: American Psychological Association.

Wolitzky, D. (2020). Contemporary Freudian psychoanalytic psychotherapy, in S. Messer & N. Kaslow (Eds.), *Essential psychotherapies* (pp. 35–70). New York: Guilford.

6   The Behavioral Paradigm

The self is… in continuous formation through choice of action.

–John Dewey

A range of intellectual traditions and philosophical perspectives have shaped
the course of understanding and practice in the behavioral paradigm over the
decades, and clinical scholars have come to encompass divergent ideas and
methods in their conceptions of therapeutic action, change, and growth. The
first generation of therapeutic approaches emerged in the 1950s, based on the
experimental psychology of behaviorism. Practitioners focused on principles of
learning and environmental conditions thought to influence overt behavior,
drawing on conceptions of classical and operant conditioning.

Following the "Cognitive Revolution" of the 1960s, a second generation of
thinkers increasingly centered on mental processes, attempting to bring mind
into the behavioral paradigm. Practitioners developed new approaches, joining
cognitive strategies and behavioral techniques in efforts to change patterns of
thinking believed to perpetuate problems in living. Over the last quarter century clinicians have continued to expand the domains of theory and practice in
elaborating third-wave models of therapy, emphasizing the crucial role of
emotion, meaning, validation, and acceptance, converging with concepts of
therapeutic action set forth in the psychoanalytic, humanistic, existential, and
Buddhist traditions. Behavioral approaches, rooted in positivism, shaped by the
scientist-practitioner tradition, have been studied more frequently than any
other form of therapy. Researchers have documented the efficacy and effectiveness of behavioral interventions for a wide range of problems in living over
the years, and they are actively promoted as empirically supported forms of
treatment, shaping models of evidence-based practice.

In this chapter I trace the emergence of the behavioral paradigm, outlining
the orienting perspectives of classical approaches, representative versions of
cognitive-behavioral therapy, and the third generation of functional and contextual models. I describe concepts of therapeutic action and illustrate the
range of approaches encompassed in the paradigm in a review of pragmatic
models that integrate ideas and methods across the three generations of practice. As in the other chapters in Part III, I consider the ways in which recent

developments in science of mind and the principles and values of clinical pragmatism enlarge our appreciation of essential concerns in behavioral conceptions of therapeutic action, change, and growth.

Origins

As we saw in the account of Freud's research as a neuroanatomist, the zeitgeist of late 19th century Europe was shaped by the emergence of empiricism, an epistemological doctrine that emphasizes the fundamental role of observation, experimentation, and evidence in the development of knowledge. Historians trace the origins of the scientific discipline of psychology to the work Wilhelm Wundt, a German researcher who established the first experimental psychology laboratory in 1879, carrying out studies of perception and psychophysics, and research on neurophysiology and behavior initiated by a series of Russian biologists, physiologists, and physicians, most notably Ivan Pavlov.

John B. Watson, a graduate of the University of Chicago, drew on these converging lines of research at the turn of the 20th century, challenging the humanistic paradigm of William James that had shaped the development of American psychology. James had taken *experience* as the starting point of his person-centered psychology, while Wundt and Watson embraced the Germanic ideal of pure scientific research. In formulating his notion of behaviorism, Watson rejected the introspective method and the study of subjectivity, emotion, consciousness, and intentionality that had served as the foundation of mentalistic theories of psychology.

Watson embraced positivism in his effort to distinguish psychology from philosophy and establish the discipline as an objective branch of natural science. In doing so he privileged materialism over mentalism, objectivity over subjectivity, and determinism over notions of free will, proposing that our behavior is governed by stimulus-response relationships. Watson's behaviorism, expanding Pavlov's research on conditioned reflexes and classical conditioning, emphasized linear models of causality, operational definition of concepts, specificity in describing relationships between variables, and quantification (Watson, 1913; see Fishman & Franks, 1997, for expanded review of the history of behavior therapy).

Subsequent thinkers, notably C. L. Hull, E. L. Thorndike, and B.F. Skinner, elaborated theories of learning through the first half of the 20th century. Thorndike introduced principles of learning and reinforcement in formulating the "law of effect" that emphasized the role of positive and negative consequences of behavior, prefiguring conceptions of operant conditioning (Thorndike, 1905). Drawing on Thorndike's contributions, Skinner elaborated basic principles of operant conditioning that informed methods of behavior modification in efforts to address problems in functioning associated with mental illness and developmental disabilities. He and his colleagues studied the use of operant conditioning strategies for treatment of behavioral problems perpetuated by psychosis at the Laboratory for Behavior Research at the

Metropolitan State Hospital in Waltham, Massachusetts, in the early 1950s. They would show how practitioners could apply the techniques of contingency management in the fields of mental health and education, introducing the term behavior therapy to describe the use of conditioning principles for a range of problems in living (Skinner, Solomon & Lindsley, 1953).

Following the fundamental tenets of behaviorism, researchers assumed that basic learning mechanisms govern our most complex behaviors, disavowing the relevance of internal mental processes. Pavlov's conceptions of classical conditioning, based on Aristotelian notions of association by contiguity, and Skinner's formulations of operant conditioning, focused on the positive or negative consequences of behavior, served as the foundation for the earliest forms of behavioral intervention.

Evolution of Therapeutic Practice

Joseph Wolpe, trained as a psychiatrist in South Africa, built on Pavlovian formulations of classical conditioning, Hull's conceptions of operant learning, and the neurology of Charles Sherrington in developing his therapeutic methods in the late 1950s, introducing counterconditioning techniques for the treatment of fear, anxiety, and avoidant behavior associated with a range of problems in living (Wolpe, 1958). Although scholars would challenge his theory of the fundamental mechanisms believed to govern change, based on neurological formulations of reciprocal inhibition, his experimental research shaped the development of exposure-based techniques in the wider domain of clinical practice. Methods of systematic desensitization, used in the treatment of fear and experiential avoidance associated with neurosis and anxiety disorders, combined methods of exposure and relaxation procedures through in-vivo engagement or visualization of anxiety-arousing situations. The repeated experience of exposure and relaxation was thought to break the associative links between stimuli and the experience of vulnerability, fear, and maladaptive behavior.

Hans Eysenck, working as a research psychologist in the Institute of Psychiatry at the University of London, also drew on the work of Pavlov and Hull in his efforts to broaden the field of behavior therapy in the 1950s. His influential critiques of psychoanalytic psychotherapy and writings on emerging developments in behavioral intervention moved clinicians to experiment with a range of procedures at the Maudsley Hospital, using conditioning and reinforcement techniques, systematic desensitization, and behavioral rehearsal (Eysenck, 1952, 1959, 1972). In his efforts to advance the application of learning theory to clinical problems, Eysenck published the first behaviorally oriented textbook on abnormal psychology in 1960, followed by collections of case studies in behavior therapy (Eysenck, 1960, 1964). He founded the first major journal devoted to behavior therapy, *Behavior research and therapy*, in 1963. The Association for the Advancement of Behavior Therapy was established three years later.

The first generation of behavior therapists continued to apply basic principles of classical and operant conditioning in their efforts to treat a variety of problems in functioning, seeking to change maladaptive emotional reactions and patterns of behavior. As clinicians engaged a wider range of concerns in community settings, however, they increasingly realized the limits of therapeutic methods based on the reductive principles of behaviorism. Critiques of the first generation of behavioral approaches documented the limits of classical learning theory and stimulus-response models of intervention that had failed to consider fundamental aspects of the mind and subjectivity, the complexities of problems in living, and the dynamics of change and growth.

Developments in the fields of cognitive science and artificial intelligence in the mid-1950s, prefiguring what we would come to know as the "Cognitive Revolution," challenged scholars to take more account of the mental processes believed to mediate our experience of emotion and behavior. Using the metaphor of the mind as a computer, researchers introduced a serial processing model of cognition that would supersede behaviorism as the orienting paradigm in the discipline of psychology.

Scholars increasingly explored the dynamics of cognition, emphasizing the crucial role of motivation, appraisal, and meaning in our experience of vulnerability, problem-solving, and coping. Albert Bandura expanded cognitive models of personality and behavior, introducing concepts of observational learning, modeling, and self-efficacy (see Bandura, 1969, 1971, 1982). Walter Mischel challenged trait theories of personality, emphasizing the ways in which contexts and situations shape different patterns of behavior (see Mischel, 1971, 1973). The ways in which we make sense of experience, create meaning, negotiate problems in living, and cope emerged as fundamental concerns in the domain of psychotherapy.

Practitioners began to integrate behavioral methods and cognitive strategies in the 1970s, introducing the first versions of cognitive-behavior therapy, taking more account of thoughts and feelings in ways that classical behavioral practitioners had failed to consider in their formulations of dysfunction, intervention, and change. Clinicians drew on the cognitive approaches of Albert Ellis and Aaron Beck, originating in clinical practice rather than in the experimental psychology of behaviorism, shaped by philosophical traditions and psychodynamic thinkers (see Chapter 7).

The emergence of the third wave of behavior therapies at the end of the 20th century reflected a radical shift in the philosophical perspectives that had shaped mechanistic conceptions of behavioral learning and serial models of cognition, moving from simplistic stimulus-response models of cause-effect relationships to non-linear, multi-causal perspectives. Scholar-practitioners increasingly acknowledged the failings of logical positivism and reductive stimulus-response models in efforts to address the complexities of problems in living, embracing a pragmatic paradigm that challenged clinicians to broaden conceptions of behavior and to explore the contexts, functions, and consequences of sensations, feelings, thoughts, and actions.

Drawing on Buddhist traditions, relational psychoanalysis, existential thought, and experiential approaches in the humanistic paradigm, practitioners introduced conceptions of acceptance, validation, and mindfulness that would help patients engage and observe—rather than attempt to control, challenge, or change—their experience of sensation, feeling, thought, imagery, and other forms of behavior that perpetuate suffering and problems in living.

From this perspective the intent is not to change the experience itself but to transform the way in which we relate to subjective states and circumstances through shifts in perspective, observing, accepting, and exploring challenging conditions without becoming overwhelmed by them. The dialectical behavior therapy of Marsha Linehan, the functional analytic psychotherapy of Robert Kohlenberg and Mavis Tsai, and the acceptance and commitment therapy of Stephen Hayes and colleagues exemplify the orienting perspectives and pragmatic concerns of the third generation, though practitioners continue to integrate concepts and strategies introduced in earlier formulations of behavior therapy. Recent developments in therapeutic practice focus on methods believed to facilitate growth across a range of diagnostic categories, moving clinical scholars to introduce "process-based" therapeutic approaches (see, for example, Barlow & Farchione, 2017; Hayes & Hoffman, 2018).

Models of Therapy

I outline three models in greater detail that illustrate the diverse forms of therapeutic action we encompass in the behavioral paradigm, exemplifying the principles and values of clinical pragmatism.

Cyclical Psychodynamics: Wachtel

Paul Wachtel has developed an integrative model of psychotherapy that bridges basic concepts and methods across the behavioral paradigm with the orienting perspectives of relational psychoanalysis, cognitive therapy, the experiential approaches of the humanistic tradition, and systemic points of view. Following his training in psychoanalysis in the 1970s, he came to appreciate the depth and complexity of understanding that had shaped psychodynamic conceptions of personality and relational life, recognizing the crucial role of unconscious processes, defenses, and conflict in our experience of vulnerability and problems in living.

In his critiques of the classical psychoanalytic paradigm, however, he argued that thinkers had overvalued early developmental experience in their formulations of vulnerability, failing to appreciate the ways in which current patterns of behavior, capacities and skills, relational life, and social surrounds perpetuate problems in living. Classical psychoanalytic thinkers had privileged "inside-out" notions of causality, focusing on concepts of developmental arrest and the dynamics of inner life, but failed to consider the influence of "outside-in" conditions that behavioral thinkers had emphasized in their formulations of problems in living, therapeutic action, learning, and change.

Drawing on the work of Walter Mischel, Wachtel increasingly realized the ways in which subjective experience and patterns of behavior vary considerably from context to context, coming to emphasize the importance of attending to the concrete particularities of what we feel, think, say and do in different situations and the variety of contingencies that shape ways of living in the present.

The *person in context* is his focal concern, and his conceptions of personality development and problems in living are based on a circular model of causality. He centers on the dynamics of "cycles of reciprocal causation between intrapsychic processes and the events of daily living," emphasizing "repetitive cycles of interactions between people" in his relational approach (Wachtel, 2011, p. 68). Inner experience and outer realities create and evoke the other through perceptual inclinations to see the old in the new and behavioral inclinations to evoke the old in the new (Wachtel, 2008, p. 104). The recursive dynamics of inner life and outer experience recreate the other. In his schema, childhood experiences are formative not because they "arrest" the development of the self but because they initiate developmental trajectories that predispose us to feel, think, and act in ways that continue to perpetuate a particular direction. In this sense the precipitants of problems in functioning lie in the interactive present, not in the distant past.

Drawing on the later work of Freud and the interpersonal perspectives of Harry Stack Sullivan and Karen Horney (see Chapters 4 and 5), he emphasizes the fundamental role of fear and anxiety in his conceptions of dysfunction, linking problems in living to "vicious circles" of feeling, thought, and behavior. Fear and anxiety create states of distress, compromising the course of development, constricting ways of being, relating, and living as one attempts to manage the continued experience of suffering. His formulations of neurosis are based on the assumption that we avoid crucial feelings, thoughts, behaviors, and situations in efforts to regulate anxiety, compromising the development of basic capacities and skills in living that require practice and shaping over the course of development.

While the function of defensive behavior is to limit the experience of vulnerability and anxiety, such protective strategies potentially generate the very psychological and interpersonal outcomes one fears, perpetuating problems in functioning. However much insight and understanding one develops about the origins of problems in living, he explains, the pattern perpetuates itself so long as one "keeps living the way he does. And he keeps living that way because he is *afraid* not to" (Wachtel, 2011, p. 74). Fear and anxiety override insight and understanding.

We carry out our life across different contexts and situations, he observes, "and our behavior, both adaptive and maladaptive, is always *in relation to* someone or something" (2011, p.77). It is crucial, accordingly, to focus on the concrete particulars of daily living, exploring the dynamics of inner life and outer realities.

In his formulations of change, shaped by Jean Piaget's conceptions of assimilation and accommodation, new behaviors produce new consequences and different feedback, which foster the development of insight, shaping subsequent patterns of feeling, thought, and action. As he emphasizes, "internal change and change in overt patterns are not really alternatives, they are two aspects of one process, and neither alone will yield reliable and satisfying results" (2011, p. 323). Change in one domain facilitates change in the other through complex feedback processes.

Over the course of psychotherapy the patient and practitioner explore the dynamics of intrapsychic life, interpersonal functioning, and contextual factors that perpetuate problems in living, clarifying maladaptive patterns of feeling, thinking, and acting that emerge in the give and take of everyday life, often recreated in the interactive experience of the therapeutic process through enactments and transference-countertransference reactions.

Drawing on concepts of classical conditioning, Wachtel assumes that one of the most powerful sources of change is direct exposure to feared aspects of inner experience (sensations, feelings, thoughts, images, memories) or actual conditions in the outer world. Methods of exposure activate, challenge, and disrupt vicious circles of feeling, thought, and action, strengthening the development of capacities and skills to deal with feared conditions. Activation of problems in functioning may occur through guided exploration of focal concerns or through enactments in patient-therapist interaction. Transference and countertransference reactions provide in-vivo opportunities for experiential learning (Wachtel, 2008, 2011).

Like third-wave behavioral practitioners, Wachtel recognizes the crucial role of acceptance and challenge in his understanding of therapeutic action, change, and growth. He outlines principles and techniques of therapeutic communication that foster the development of capacities and skills through experiential learning in the clinical situation. He makes pragmatic use of a range of behavioral concepts and procedures over the course of treatment, including in-vivo exposure and systematic desensitization, relaxation techniques, modeling, role-playing, skills training, and planned activities in the surrounds of everyday life.

Deepened understanding and insight are crucial in helping patients strengthen their sense of personal agency and the "experience of oneself as the vital center giving direction to daily actions and choices" (2011, p. 102). In accordance with behavioral conceptions of change, however, Wachtel emphasizes the crucial functions of *action* and experiential learning in the outer world. Over the course of the therapeutic process patients strengthen capacities and skills that have been compromised by fear, avoidance, and restrictions of opportunity, and engage the experience of living more fully and deeply in the present (for expanded accounts see Wachtel, 2014).

Dialectical Behavior Therapy: Linehan

Marsha Linehan introduced the first version of dialectical behavior therapy in 1993 as an integrative approach for the treatment of problems in functioning associated with borderline personality disorder. Drawing on relational concepts from the humanistic paradigm, she emphasized the crucial role of the therapeutic alliance and the clinician's validation of the patient's experience in change and growth. She integrated core concepts and methods of behavioral intervention based on the principles of classical conditioning and operant learning, including exposure, contingency management, and skills training, and fundamental elements of Zen Buddhism and the practice of mindfulness, which emphasizes the radical acceptance and validation of experience without attempting to change it. Linehan came to think of the approach as a behavioral treatment program, encompassing individual psychotherapy, skills training, telephone coaching, and peer consultation.

Linehan centers on the paradoxical dynamics of acceptance and change in her dialectical conceptions of therapeutic action. In the course of her practice she came to believe that traditional cognitive behavioral models of intervention, emphasizing the process of change, potentially invalidate the patient's subjective experience and sense of reality, intensifying arousal, compromising cognitive function and coping capacities.

Drawing on the principles of Buddhist thought, she introduced perspectives and practices that would help patients strengthen their capacities to accept, tolerate, and validate inner experience and outer realities rather than attempt to avoid, challenge, or change them. She integrated mindfulness meditation in efforts to help patients engage the experience of the present, accepting the flow of sensations, feelings, thoughts, and images without judgement or attempting to change inner states. The clinician reaffirms the ways in which the patient's feelings, thoughts, and actions make sense in light of earlier experience and current circumstances.

While methods of validation foster the experience of acceptance, problem-solving strategies focus on change. In this sense the approach seeks to foster a synthesis between alternative positions in light of changing needs, capacities, and circumstances. The therapist carries out a functional analysis of behavior, exploring the antecedents and consequences of feelings, thoughts, and actions, considering a variety of approaches in light of changing needs, capacities, and circumstances, encompassing methods of exposure, contingency management, skills training, behavioral rehearsal, and cognitive restructuring. The model includes educational strategies that help patients strengthen skills in emotional regulation, distress tolerance, mindfulness meditation, and interpersonal effectiveness.

Linehan describes four stages of therapy in her efforts to address the range of problems in functioning associated with borderline personality disorder. In broad outline, the first stage focuses on patterns of behavior that potentially threaten life, compromise quality of life, or limit capacities to make use of help and care in the clinical situation. The second stage strengthens capacities to experience and process the dynamics of emotion through methods of exposure and acceptance. The third stage centers on the development of capacities and skills that facilitate efforts to pursue life goals in light of essential concerns, values, and purposes. The fourth stage, emphasizing the practice of mindfulness, seeks to deepen capacities for meaning and fulfillment.

Although the model is carefully structured, the approach is idiographic, focused on the particular circumstances of the clinical situation. If the patient has not developed the skills needed to negotiate current challenges and problems in living, for example, the therapist assumes an educational role, creating opportunities for instruction and practice. If the patient is unable to make use of capacities because of emotional dysregulation, the therapist attempts to help the patient restore stability through methods of exposure and mindfulness practice that strengthen tolerance of distress (Linehan, 1993; Linehan & Dexter-Mazza, 2008).

In a recent account of her work, Linehan describes the approach as "pragmatic, down-to-earth therapy... a program of self-improvement" (2020, p. 172). In accord with the values of clinical pragmatism, she emphasizes the "egalitarian relationship" between the therapist and the patient (2020, p. 168).

Acceptance and Commitment Therapy: Hayes and Colleagues

The acceptance and commitment therapy of Stephen Hayes and colleagues, developed over the last quarter century, provides a radical alternative to traditional behavioral approaches centered on the treatment of symptoms associated with specific disorders, challenging patients to develop capacities and skills instrumental in their efforts to pursue goals in accord with fundamental values, concerns, and purposes.

Working as a scientist-practitioner in the behavioral tradition, Hayes created the approach for patients who find themselves unable to change the content of feelings, thoughts, and actions that perpetuate problems in living. The therapeutic process seeks to help patients reinterpret the meaning of their subjective experience by creating new contexts of understanding, shifting the ways in which they relate to sensations, feelings, thoughts, and images, moving toward valued behavior and outcomes. In this sense the approach converges with existential concerns in the psychoanalytic and humanistic paradigms of psychotherapy.

He assumes that a range of problems in functioning originate in experiential avoidance, vicious circles of cognition, and patterns of rigidity that limit capacities to act in accordance with essential concerns, values, and goals. Problems in functioning that appear uncontrollable or distressing in one context become different phenomena in another context, Hayes proposes, explaining: "By establishing a posture of psychological acceptance, events that formerly were taken to be inherently problematic become instead opportunities for growth, interest, or understanding" (Hayes, 1994, p. 13). The goal is to help patients strengthen capacities to engage, experience, and observe the dynamics of inner life, working to strengthen agency and pursue goals in the service of growth and individuation.

Hayes thinks of behaviors as *acts in context*, evaluated by their effectiveness in bringing about outcomes that foster flexibility, change, and growth. He enlarges conceptions of behavior to encompass the dynamics of cognition and the symbolic meaning of language, drawing on Skinner's philosophy of radical behaviorism, focusing on the functions of verbal behavior.

The functional analysis of behavior clarifies the antecedents (discriminative stimuli), focal behaviors (response repertoire), and consequences (contingencies of reinforcement). The expanded conceptions of behavior allow practitioners to move beyond the realm of observable, overt events and explore the functional relationships among the *meanings* of behavioral antecedents and their consequences.

Formulations of therapeutic action, based on the principles of classical and operant conditioning, encompass a range of approaches and methods in efforts to alter the variables that precipitate problems in living and shape the contingencies of reinforcement in accord with the patient's values and commitments. Practitioners seek to strengthen the development of capacities for presence, acceptance, clarification of values, and commitment to action in light of fundamental concerns and goals. The core principles of change and growth emphasize engagement of the present moment (awareness of here and now experience approached with openness, interest, and curiosity); the attitude of acceptance (embracing the flow of sensations, feelings, thoughts, images and memories without judgment or challenge); cognitive defusion (challenging tendencies to reify thoughts, feelings, images, and memories); clarification of values and purposes; and commitments to action in constructive efforts to develop capacities and achieve goals.

Therapeutic Action

As we have seen, the behavioral paradigm challenges us to focus on the concrete particularities of the clinical situation, centering on immediate concerns, exploring what our patients feel, think, do, and want, and clarifying the dynamics of specific processes and the nature of concrete conditions thought to perpetuate problems in functioning. From the behavioral point of view, as we have seen, the self is "in continuous formation through *choice of action*," as Dewey proposed (1916, p. 408).

Clinical scholars continue to emphasize notions of learning in their formulations of what is the matter and what carries the potential to help, drawing on concepts of capability, mastery, and growth. We have learned ways of dealing with particular situations that now limit us, presumably, and the fundamental aim of intervention is to help us learn more functional ways of negotiating concerns, coping with problems in living, and strengthening capacities and skills.

We consider the role of context, language, meaning, values, action, experiential learning, and the development of skills in our formulations of therapeutic action, change, and growth. Wachtel documents the growing emphasis on emotion, acceptance, and validation in his accounts of the behavioral paradigm, emphasizing the experiential character of therapeutic methods that foster efforts to learn by doing, strengthening capacities and skills (Wachtel, 1997, 2011).

In contrast to classical models of behavioral treatment that had focused largely on technical procedures, contemporary practitioners increasingly recognize the crucial role of the therapeutic alliance and the collaborative nature of intervention in accord with the principles and values of clinical pragmatism. Therapists and patients explore the concrete particulars of current concerns, working to clarify the contexts, antecedents, dynamics, and consequences of feelings, thoughts, and actions that perpetuate problems in living.

From the perspective of the behavioral paradigm, what we feel, think, say, and do varies from situation to situation, shaped by changing contexts and circumstances, and practitioners focus on specific patterns of stimulus and response across the relationships, activities, and surrounds of everyday life.

Following the fundamental principles of operant conditioning, clinicians assume that the consequences of behaviors increase or decrease the likelihood that particular patterns of feeling, thinking, and acting will recur. In carrying out the functional analysis of behavior, accordingly, practitioners and patients carefully explore the outcomes of feelings, thoughts, and actions associated with problems in living, taking account of the contexts of focal concerns and the contingencies thought to reinforce maladaptive patterns of functioning. The goal of the analysis is to identify specific stimuli that activate problematic forms of behavior, factors that reinforce dysfunctional patterns, and conditions that strengthen the development of capacities, skills, and adaptive outcomes. Clinicians draw on conceptions of reinforcement, extinction, shaping, and practice in structuring the course and activities of intervention (Antony, Roemer & Lenton-Brym, 2020).

Psychotherapists across the foundational schools of thought continue to recognize the role of operant conditioning in change and growth, broadening concepts of therapeutic action to take account of crucial sources of reinforcement operating in the core conditions of the relationship and the dynamics of interactive experience as well as contingencies that shape behavior in the ongoing relationships, activities, and surrounds of everyday life, often neglected in case formulations (see Wachtel, 1997, for discussion of contingencies that reinforce behavior in the clinical situation and everyday life).

Clinicians have come to appreciate the powerful influence of exposure in efforts to address a range of problems in functioning, introducing a variety of methods that help patients negotiate the experience of fear and avoidance. Patients engage anxiety-arousing situations in real life through in-vivo forms of exposure. Focused exploration of the dynamics of inner life and imaginal approaches in the therapeutic process help patients generate the experience of feelings, thoughts, and memories that they perceive as threatening. Interoceptive modes of exposure allow patients to recreate the visceral experience of feared sensations through different forms of activity that engage physiological processes instrumental in the distressing reactions (for reviews of exposure methods see Anthony, Roemer & Lenton-Brym, 2020; Barlow, 2004; and Wachtel, 1997, 2011).

Eye movement desensitization and reprocessing (EMDR), developed by Francine Shapiro, is a version of exposure therapy that employs imaginal flooding and cognitive restructuring in efforts to help patients process and integrate traumatic experience (Shapiro, 2017). The approach, using rapid, rhythmic eye movements and other forms of bilateral stimulation, encompasses a range of behavioral procedures.

In contrast to traditional concepts of therapeutic action set forth in the psychodynamic and humanistic paradigms, behaviorally oriented practitioners often use structured activities and tasks in efforts to help patients develop capacities and skills through experiential learning.

Over the course of the therapeutic process the clinician may model effective ways of dealing with particular situations, engage the patient in role-play of anticipated circumstances, or provide structured opportunities for the development and practice of behaviors within the sessions. Skills training approaches focused on communication, social interaction, assertive behavior, and problem-solving have been developed for the treatment of problems in living associated with a range of conditions, including schizophrenia, depression, anxiety disorders, and stress-related disorders. The clinician functions as an educator, consultant, or role model, providing information, instruction, and feedback.

Methods of behavioral activation, originally developed for the treatment of depression, challenge extended periods of inactivity, withdrawal, and avoidance associated with a range of conditions that limit opportunities to generate enriching experience and engage positive sources of reinforcement. The therapist and patient carry out a functional analysis of behavior and collaborate in efforts to plan tasks and re-regulate patterns of activity in the routine of everyday life.

Practitioners have expanded concepts of therapeutic action in third-wave models of therapy, as noted earlier, increasingly emphasizing the attitude of acceptance, validation, meaning, values, and mindfulness practices. The goal is to help patients engage rather than avoid, challenge, or judge the dynamics of inner life that perpetuate problems in functioning. Patients focus on sensation, emotion, thought, imagery, or memory in an active experience of observation, exploration, and acceptance.

Over the decades researchers have demonstrated the efficacy and effectiveness of behavioral interventions for a wide range of disorders and problems in living. Although a review of the empirical literature is beyond the scope of this chapter, researchers have provided carefully focused accounts of studies and meta-analyses (see Antony, Roemer & Lenton-Brym, 2020; Hoffman, Asnaani, Vonk, Sawyer & Fang, 2012; Nathan & Gorman, 2014).

Although clinicians in the evidence-based practice movement continue to embrace nomothetic models of therapy, using standardized protocols for the treatment of specific symptoms associated with particular diagnostic categories, surveys show that most behaviorally oriented practitioners take an idiographic approach to intervention, making flexible use of a range of ideas and methods in light of the particular circumstances of the clinical situation (Antony, Roemer & Lenton-Brym, 2020). David Barlow distinguishes "psychological treatments," or subgroups of technical procedures focused on treatment of specific symptoms associated with particular mental disorders, from broader conceptions of psychotherapy intended to address a wider range of concerns and problems in living (Barlow, 2004).

From the perspective of clinical pragmatism, as noted earlier, practitioners may combine technical procedures developed in standardized treatment protocols with ideas and methods from other schools of thought over the course of psychotherapy. As we will see in the case reports presented in Chapter 9, behavioral concepts and methods lend themselves to applications in integrative approaches across the foundational schools of thought (for further reviews of assessment procedures and methods of intervention see Anthony, Roemer & Lenton-Brym, 2020; Wachtel, 1997).

Neuroscience and Therapeutic Action

As emphasized in earlier accounts of neuroscience and attachment, clinical scholars propose that the interactive experience of the therapeutic process carries the potential to activate bonding processes associated with neuroplasticity, strengthening capacities to process subjective experience, regulate sensation and emotion, engage relational life, and initiate activities that sponsor change and growth. Although conceptions of therapeutic action in traditional models of behavioral and cognitive-behavioral intervention have emphasized technical procedures rather than the core conditions and functions of the therapeutic relationship, as discussed earlier, the second and third generations of practitioners have increasingly recognized the crucial role of the therapeutic alliance, collaboration, and the dynamics of interactive experience. Clinicians have reformulated psychodynamic and humanistic accounts of relational experience from a behavioral perspective, emphasizing concepts of acceptance, validation, and reinforcement.

Researchers assume that moderate arousal or "optimal stress" fosters neuroplasticity, learning, change, and growth, as outlined in Chapter 2. A variety of methods and activities encompassed in the behavioral paradigm carry the potential to intensify the experience of emotion, challenging patients to engage, embody, tolerate, and accept sensations, feelings, thoughts, images, and memories associated with fear, avoidance, and problems in living, creating conditions thought to activate the production of neurotransmitters and hormones instrumental in long-term potentiation, neural integration, and cortical reorganization.

As we have seen, behavioral thinkers continue to focus on the dynamics of association in formulations of learning, change, and growth, centering on the relationships between stimuli, responses, and reinforcing conditions. Associative connections are strengthened by their repeated conjunction, in reality or in imagination.

Over the years, practitioners have elaborated different methods of exposure and desensitization believed to challenge and weaken the associative links between stimuli and responses, fostering the reorganization of neural networks, strengthening capacities to regulate emotion. Methods of behavioral activation and skills training help patients challenge the inertia and avoidance associated with a range of problems in functioning, likely to generate moderate levels of stress associated with neuroplasticity.

Beyond the experiential opportunities of the therapeutic process itself, clinicians have encompassed a wide range of methods and activities in their efforts to help patients *act* in the course of everyday life, initiating new patterns of behavior in the outer world, including skills training, structured tasks, and planned activities. Some clinicians combine traditional behavioral methods of intervention with "bottom-up" practices believed to engage subcortical regions of the brain, including relaxation techniques, mindfulness meditation, music, dance, tai chi, and other forms of activity that use physical movement and breath, reregulating physiological states and emotion. Drawing on converging lines of study in the fields of neuroscience and trauma, researchers urge clinicians to expand the range of therapeutic approaches that engage the domains of sensation, emotion, action, and movement, hopeful that more bodily oriented forms of intervention will offer the possibility of "reprogramming" automatic physical reactions that perpetuate problems in functioning (see Van der Kolk, 2014, p. 168).

Concluding Comments

As we have seen, the earliest versions of behavioral treatment emerged from the epistemological doctrine of empiricism, based on concepts of classical and operant conditioning, disavowing the relevance of mental constructs and subjective experience, treating thoughts and feelings as epiphenomena. Over time, researchers and practitioners engaged a wider range of ideas, expanding the scope of theory and practice in more complex versions of cognitive-behavior therapy and third-wave models of treatment.

Contemporary thinkers have come to embrace pragmatic philosophy as an alternative to the mechanistic worldview that had shaped earlier approaches, viewing behavior as "acts in context," focusing on the functional relations and consequences of sensations, feelings, thoughts and actions, judging ideas and methods by their outcomes—what practical difference they make in the concrete particularities of everyday life (see Follette & Callaghan, 2011; Hayes & Hoffman, 2018; and Masuda & Rizvi, 2020, for discussion of pragmatic philosophy and the orienting perspectives of third-wave behavioral therapy). The pragmatic paradigm rejects the search for general laws that had shaped the experimental psychology of behaviorism, focusing on the particular experience of the whole person in context (see Masuda & Rizvi, 2020, for an expanded discussion of "elemental realism" and "functional contextualism" in the behavioral paradigm).

Emerging models of therapeutic action, emphasizing flexible use of ideas and methods in idiographic, "process-based" approaches to help and care, engage essential concerns in the formulations of clinical pragmatism outlined here. Clinicians center on the subjectivity of the individual, taking account of values, meaning, commitments, and goals; the crucial role of the therapeutic relationship, collaboration, use of interactive experience, and methods of communication; and the fundamental importance of action and experiential learning in understanding, change, and growth—*learning by doing*, as Dewey emphasizes in his pragmatic philosophy.

Reference

Antony, M., Roemer, L. & Lenton-Brym, A. (2020). Behavior therapy: Traditional approaches, in S. Messer & N. Kaslow (Eds.), *Essential psychotherapies*, 4th edn (pp. 111–141). New York: Guilford.

Bandura, A. (1969). *Principles of behavior modification*. New York: Holt, Rinehart and Winston.

Bandura, A. (1971). Psychotherapy based upon modeling principles, in A. E. Bergin & S. L. Garfield (Eds.), *Handbook of psychotherapy and behavior change* (pp. 653–708). New York: Wiley.

Bandura, A. (1982). Self efficacy mechanism in human agency. *American Psychologist*, 37, 122–147.

Barlow, D. (2004). Psychological treatments. *American Psychologist*, 59, 869–878.

Barlow, D. & Farchione, T. J. (2017). *Applications of the unified protocol for transdiagnostic treatment of emotional disorders*. New York: Oxford University Press.

Dewey, J. (1916). *Democracy and education: An introduction to the philosophy of education*. New York: Macmillan

Eysenck, H. (1952). The effects of psychotherapy: An evaluation. *Journal of Consulting Psychology*, 16, 319–324.

Eysenck, H. (1959). Learning theory and behavior therapy. *Journal of Mental Science*, 105, 61–75.

Eysenck, H. (1960). *Handbook of abnormal psychology: An experimental approach*. London: Pitman.

Eysenck, H. (Ed.) (1964). *Experiments in behavior therapy: Readings in modern methods of treating mental disorders derived from learning theory*. Elmsford, NY: Pergamon Press.

Eysenck, H. (1972). Behavior therapy is behavioristic. *Behavior Therapy*, 3, 609–613.

Fishman, D. & Franks, C. (1997). The conceptual evolution of behavior therapy, in P. Wachtel & S. Messer (Eds.), *Theories of psychotherapy* (pp. 131–169). Washington, DC: American Psychological Association.

Follette, W. & Callaghan, G. (2011). Behavior therapy: Functional and contextual perspectives, in S. Messer & A. Gurman (Eds.), *Essential psychotherapies*, 3rd edn (pp. 184–222). New York: Guilford.

Hayes, S. C. (1994). Content, context, and the types of psychological acceptance, in S. C. Hayes, N. S. Jacobson, V. Follette & M. J. Dougher (Eds.), *Acceptance and change: Content and context in psychotherapy* (pp. 13–32). Reno, NV: Context Press.

Hayes, S. C. & Hoffman, S. G. (2018). *Process-based CBT: The science and core clinical competencies of cognitive behavioral therapy*. Reno, NV: Context Press.

Hoffman, S., Asnaani, A., Vonk, K. J., Sawyer, A. T. & Fang, A. (2012). The efficacy of cognitive behavioral therapy: A review of meta-analyses. *Cognitive Therapy Research*, 36, 427–440.

Linehan, M. (1993). *Cognitive-behavioral treatment of borderline personality disorder.* New York: Guilford.

Linehan, M. (2020). *Building a life worth living.* New York: Random House.

Linehan, M. & Dexter-Mazza, E. (2008). Dialectical behavior therapy for borderline personality disorder, in D. Barlow (Ed.), *Clinical handbook for psychiatric disorders* (pp. 365–420). New York: Guilford.

Masuda, A. & Rizvi, S. (2020). Third-wave cognitive-behaviorally based therapies, in S. Messer & N. Kaslow (Eds.). *Essential psychotherapies*, 4th edn (pp. 183–220). New York: Guilford.

Mischel, W. (1971). *Introduction to personality.* New York: Holt, Rinehart & Winston.

Mischel, W. (1973). Toward a cognitive social learning reconceptualization of personality. *Psychological Review*, 80, 252–283.

Nathan, P. & Gorman, J. (Eds.) (2014). *A guide to treatments that work*, 4th edn. New York: Oxford University Press.

Shapiro, F. (2017). *Eye movement desensitization and reprocessing (EMDR) therapy*, 3rd edn. New York: Guilford.

Skinner, B. F., Solomon, C. & Lindsley, O. R. (1953). *Studies in behavior therapy: Status Report 1* (Unpublished report). Waltham, MA: Metropolitan State Hospital.

Thorndike, E. L. (1905). *The elements of psychology.* New York: A.G. Seiler.

Van der Kolk, B. (2014). Clinical implications of neuroscience research in PTSD, in G. Leo (Ed.), *Neuroscience and psychoanalysis* (pp. 159–196). Lecce, Italy: Frenis Zero Press.

Wachtel, P. (1997). *Psychoanalysis, behavior therapy, and the relational world.* Washington, DC: American Psychological Association.

Wachtel, P. (2008). *Relational theory and the practice of psychotherapy.* New York: Guilford.

Wachtel, P. (2011). *Therapeutic communication*, 2nd edn. New York: Guilford.

Wachtel, P. (2014). *Cyclical psychodynamics and the contextual self.* New York: Routledge.

Watson, J. (1913). Psychology as the behaviorist views it. *Psychological Review*, 20, 158–177.

Wolpe, J. (1958). *Psychotherapy by reciprocal inhibition.* Stanford, CA: Stanford University Press.

7   The Cognitive Paradigm

> ... whatever elements an act of cognition may imply... it at least implies the existence of a feeling.
>
> –William James

Over the last quarter century critiques and reformulations of cognitive therapy have brought about major shifts in understanding and practice. Although the earliest versions of treatment privileged a rationalist epistemology and objectivist conceptions of truth, exemplified in the classical approaches of Albert Ellis and Aaron Beck, contemporary models have increasingly come to emphasize the active properties of mind and the constructive nature of knowing. Over the course of development we establish mental structures or schemata that mediate our experience of emotion, meaning, and behavior, encompassing what we understand as our assumptive worlds, beliefs and attitudes, personal narratives, and patterns of thought.

The growing emphasis on emotion, meaning, and the social surround has enlarged the scope of cognitive therapy, and recent approaches converge with developments in the science of mind, psychodynamic thought, narrative psychology, Buddhist conceptions of mindfulness, and third-wave behavioral models of intervention. Following moves toward integrative practice in the broader field of psychotherapy, clinicians continue to make use of ideas and methods across the foundational schools of thought in their efforts to address a wider range of problems in living and to take more account of conditions and circumstances in the social surround that perpetuate vulnerability. Over the decades researchers have documented the efficacy and effectiveness of cognitive approaches for a range of problems in living, and they are actively promoted as empirically supported forms of therapy, shaping models of evidence-based practice.

In this chapter I trace the emergence of the cognitive paradigm and explore the ways in which concepts of therapeutic action in classical and contemporary approaches deepen our understanding of core processes believed to bring about change and growth. As a starting point I review the intellectual traditions that have shaped the development of the paradigm. I outline the evolution of clinical practice in the next section, reviewing concepts of therapeutic action, and describe a series of models that exemplify the range of concerns and methods encompassed in the paradigm. As in the other chapters in Part III, I consider the ways in which recent developments in the science of mind and the principles and values of clinical pragmatism deepen our appreciation of essential concerns in conceptions of therapeutic action, change, and growth.

Origins

A range of intellectual traditions in philosophy, psychology, and Buddhist thought have shaped the development of cognitive perspectives in therapeutic practice. Scholars trace the origins of fundamental assumptions to the writings of classical Greek and Roman philosophers, often citing the epigram of the 4th century Stoic thinker Epictetus, "we are not disturbed by events, but by the views we take of them." As Henri Ellenberger, the historian of depth psychology, explains: "The element of psychic training was stressed among the Stoics and the Epicureans. The Stoics learned the control of emotions and practiced written and verbal exercises in concentration and meditation" (Ellenberger, 1970, p. 42).

A series of European philosophers, prefiguring contemporary constructivist perspectives, came to think of knowledge as an active structuring of experience, emphasizing the transformative properties of mind. Giambattista Vico, the Italian rhetorician, proposed that we make sense of the world through linguistic abstractions, myths, and fables. Immanuel Kant argued that the mind organizes and orders the phenomena of experience, anticipating contemporary formulations of schemata. Hans Vaihinger, a Kant scholar, introduced the philosophy of "as if," believing that we develop "workable fictions" in order to pursue organizing purposes and goals. Ernst Cassirer explored the ways in which symbolic and linguistic constructs shape our experience of the world. Jean Piaget, influenced by Kant's notion of innate categories, centered on the role of dynamic learning in the creation of meaning in fashioning his model of cognitive development. George Kelly drew on the work of Vaihinger in developing his theory of "personal constructs." Postmodern thinkers have expanded constructivist and narrative perspectives, seeing the viability of any given meaning as a function of its practical consequences for the individual in the concrete particularity of historical, social, and cultural surrounds (see Borden, 2010; Messer & Wachtel, 1997).

In the psychodynamic paradigm, as we have seen, classical and contemporary thinkers have explored cognitive processes in their formulations of personality, vulnerability, and psychotherapy. Freud described the organization and structure of memory and introduced an early version of cognitive psychology in his accounts of the mind, exploring the relationship between conscious and unconscious domains of motivation, thought, and emotion in his theories of personality, psychopathology, and therapeutic action (see Erdelyi, 1985; Kandel, 2012; and Wakefield & Baer, 2010, for accounts of Freudian thought and cognitive psychology).

In developing his theory of psychological types, C. G. Jung outlined what he regarded as basic modes of information processing, broadly categorized as thinking, feeling, sensing, and intuiting, encompassing what we would now recognize as core functions of the right and left hemispheres of the brain. Alfred Adler came to think of consciousness as the center of personality, and emphasized the role of perception, cognition, learning, and meaning in elaborating his relational perspective; he is increasingly characterized as a constructivist thinker, prefiguring the emergence of cognitive therapy.

In the interpersonal school of thought, Harry Stack Sullivan emphasized cognitive processes in his formulations of defense, such as "selective inattention," and Karen Horney described "vicious circles" of thought, feeling, and behavior that perpetuate problems in living. In the domain of object relations psychology, W. R. D. Fairbairn and John Bowlby explored the ways we internalize elements of relational life and develop schemata or "working models" that shape ways of processing interpersonal experience and patterns of behavior.

Experimental research in the fields of cognitive neuroscience and cognitive psychology continues to document the ways in which unconscious networks of association influence feelings, thoughts, and actions out of awareness, bridging basic science and reformulations of implicit processes in contemporary psychoanalysis (Schore, 2019a, 2019b; Siegel, 2020; Westen, 2005).

As noted in the previous chapter, critiques of behavior therapy, originating in the Cognitive Revolution of the 1950s, explored the limits of classical learning theory and stimulus-response models of intervention that had failed to consider the dynamics of mental life and subjective experience. Clinical scholars increasingly focused on cognitive processes, emphasizing the crucial role of appraisal and meaning in the experience of vulnerability and reactions to stressful events. Albert Bandura and Walter Mischel centered on the role of cognition, mastery, and self-efficacy in expanding conceptions of personality and change in psychotherapy, bridging essential concerns in the behavioral and cognitive traditions. Scholars increasingly explored the dynamics of coping and adaptation, emphasizing the interdependence of physiological, emotional, cognitive, and behavioral processes (see, for example, Lazarus & Folkman, 1984).

Tenzin Gyatso, the 14th Dalai Lama, came to think of Buddhism as a "science of mind" (2005), and clinical scholars have drawn on fundamental elements of Buddhist thought in their efforts to expand concepts of therapeutic action in cognitive and cognitive-behavioral models of treatment. As we find in the psychodynamic, behavioral, and humanistic paradigms, clinical approaches integrate Buddhist notions of suffering and compassion, radical acceptance of self and the desire for change, and basic methods of mindfulness training (for expanded accounts see Batchelor, 2017; Dowd & McClearly, 2007; Epstein, 2018; Siegel, 2020; and Wright, 2017).

Evolution of Therapeutic Practice

Albert Ellis and Aaron Beck, originally trained as psychoanalysts, introduced the earliest versions of cognitive therapy in the second half of the 20th century, and their approaches exemplify the defining features of what scholars have come to call the rationalist paradigm.

Ellis, influenced by the writings of the Stoic philosophers, Kant, Bertrand Russell, and Karl Popper and the psychodynamic perspectives of Alfred Adler, Karen Horney, and Eric Fromm, began to formulate his model of rational-emotive therapy in the late 1950s. He theorized that neurotic patterns of behavior originate in irrational beliefs about life events. He assumed that we learn irrational patterns of thinking over the course of our development and continue to recreate dysfunctional ways of thinking that perpetuate problems in living. He proposed that we filter our perceptions through the distorted beliefs and ideas we hold about ourselves and our experience rather than negotiating actual events in a rational, objective manner.

In his didactic approach, concepts of therapeutic action emphasize education and persuasion. The therapist is active, using rhetoric, challenge, and modeling in efforts to help patients identify and refute irrational beliefs, generate new forms of behavior, and work toward a more rational, functional philosophy of life. Ellis emphasizes the crucial role of thinking and action rather than expression of emotion in his formulations of change and growth (Ellis, 1962; Ellis & Bernard, 1985).

Beck is widely regarded as the principal architect of modern cognitive therapy. His approach originated in research on depression that he began to carry out in the late 1950s as a psychiatrist at the University of Pennsylvania. He challenged psychoanalytic conceptions of depression that had focused largely on concepts of motivation and emotion and began to explore the role of cognitive processes in the illness experience, focusing on the form and content of negative thinking.

Drawing on his clinical experience, he came to think of cognitive distortion as a defining feature of depressive syndromes, proposing that cognitive processes mediate dysfunctional patterns of feeling and behavior. The task of therapy, accordingly, is to deepen our awareness of implicit cognitive processes, explicitly formulate maladaptive thoughts, and restructure core beliefs and schemata in light of actual circumstances and realistic prospects. Although Beck built on Ellis' framework in developing his model, he found himself uncomfortable with his authoritarian style, coming to emphasize the importance of the therapeutic alliance and a "collaborative empiricism" over the course of experiential learning.

In accord with the basic assumptions of the rationalist paradigm, Ellis and Beck believed that cognitive processes organize and govern our functioning. Health, well-being, and adaptive outcomes depend on our capacities for empirical observation, rationality, hypothesis testing, and learning.

Jerome Bruner reconceptualized mind as a creator of meaning in his powerful critique of the "Cognitive Revolution," rejecting the mechanistic models of information processing that had shaped understanding in neuroscience and psychology, exploring the ways in which we render experience into words and construct stories that shape our sense of self, relational life, and culture (Bruner, 1990). Influenced by developments in narrative psychology and postmodern thought, clinical scholars began to introduce constructivist formulations of cognitive therapy toward the end of the 20th century, challenging the rationalist epistemology that had shaped the original versions of treatment. Thinkers embraced phenomenological, narrative, relational, and experiential perspectives, exploring the ways in which we create worlds of meaning and construct our experience of self, others, and reality. States of mind are mediated by our experience of emotion and constructive symbolic processes from this post-rationalist perspective. We speak not of a universal, objective reality but of multiple realities, returning to William James' notion of a "multiverse."

Michael Mahoney, Vittorio Guidano, Robert Neimeyer, and Donald Meichenbaum drew on a range of intellectual traditions in elaborating constructivist models of therapy, including the philosophical writings of Heraclitus, Kant, Vico, Schopenhauer, and Vaihinger; the cognitive psychology of Lev Vygotsky, Piaget, and Kelly; the narrative and existential perspectives of Adler and Victor Frankl; and orienting concepts in Buddhist thought (see Mahoney, 1995, 2003, 2004; Mahoney & Granvold, 2005; Meichenbaum, 2017; Neimeyer, 2009).

They enlarged the scope of the cognitive paradigm, exploring the realm of the body and the dynamics of interoceptive experience, the regulation of inner states, and the ways in which unconscious emotional and cognitive processes mediate our perceptions of experience and patterns of meaning. They challenged the emphasis on technique that had guided rationalist models of therapeutic action, offering an orienting philosophy and basic principles of practice rather than specific sequences or methods of intervention.

The constructivist thinkers centered on the crucial functions of the therapeutic relationship and the dynamics of interactive experience in their conceptions of change and growth, converging with humanistic approaches outlined in Chapter 8. In contrast to the analytical, didactic, rhetorical style that had characterized the models of Ellis and Beck, they emphasized the egalitarian and collaborative nature of the relationship and the crucial functions of ongoing dialogue, seeking to strengthen capacities for personal agency and the process of experiencing: "We are agents that act on and in the world," Mahoney wrote, joining notions of experiential learning, knowing, and self-efficacy that had shaped Dewey's account of pragmatic philosophy: "the individual is considered to be the active agent in the process of experiencing" (Mahoney & Granvold, 2005, p. 76).

Therapists explored the phenomenal world of the patient, arguing that we cannot presume to know the "truth" of the matter or serve as the arbiter of reality. The practitioner and the patient are co-creators, re-formulating accounts of life experience in efforts to sponsor coping, adaptation, and growth (Meichenbaum, 1995, p. 149).

From the perspective of the constructivist approach, the therapeutic project is centered on the dialectic between acceptance of the patient's experience and efforts to challenge features of the assumptive world, thought, and meaning that perpetuate vulnerability and problems in living. As Paul Wachtel explains, the task is not to persuade the patient that one's ways of thinking, feeling, and acting are irrational or incorrect, but to deepen understanding of the ways in which one has come to perceive circumstances and render experience, to consider the practical consequences of these interpretations, and to explore other readings that sponsor more functional ways of attending, understanding, and acting (Wachtel, 1997, 2011).

Although the constructivist thinkers de-emphasized the role of technique in their formulations of the therapeutic process, they drew on ideas and methods across the foundational schools of thought in accord with the pluralist orientation of clinical pragmatism, varying ways of working in light of changing needs, tasks, and the outcomes of experiential learning. In this sense the constructivist approaches prefigured the trend toward integrative practice in the wider cognitive paradigm as clinicians continued to join ideas and methods from psychodynamic, behavioral, and humanistic points of view. Jeremy Safran combined concepts from relational psychoanalysis, research on emotion, and cognitive methods in expanding concepts of therapeutic action (1998). Shortly after the turn of the century Sharon Berlin introduced an integrative model that bridged rationalist and constructivist approaches with contextual and systemic perspectives (Berlin, 2002, 2010).

Buddhist psychology and mindfulness practices have continued to influence the development of integrative approaches in the cognitive paradigm. In contrast to traditional versions of treatment that emphasize challenge and change, mindfulness approaches focus on observation and acceptance of inner experience. Patients follow the flow of sensations, feelings, thoughts, and images as they emerge, without judgment or attempts to avoid, escape or control them, embracing an attitude of acceptance. Clinical scholars propose that the skills of attentional control developed in mindfulness training bring about changes in patterns of thinking and attitudes toward sensations, feelings, and thoughts, viewing them as transitory phenomena rather than as full reflections of reality. The "mindfulness-based stress reduction" program developed by Jon Kabat-Zinn and the "mindfulness-based cognitive therapy" created by Zindel Segal, Mark Williams, and John Teasdale converge with essential concerns in the third-wave behavioral models of intervention reviewed in Chapter 6 (Kabat-Zinn, 2013; Segal, Williams & Teasdale, 2013).

Models of Cognitive Therapy

In this section I outline a series of models in greater detail that illustrate the diverse conceptions of therapeutic action we encompass in rationalist, constructivist, and integrative versions of intervention in the cognitive paradigm.

Rationalist Model: Beck

Aaron Beck's model of cognitive therapy is widely regarded as the exemplar of the rationalist paradigm, and his formulations have influenced concepts of therapeutic action across the foundational schools of thought (DeRubeis, Keefe & Beck, 2019). Although the approach originated in his research on depression, he developed protocols to address a wider range of symptoms and disorders over the course of his research and practice, integrating approaches from the behavioral paradigm, including methods of exposure, activation, social skills training, and relaxation procedures.

In formulating his cognitive model of depression, he distinguished three levels of cognition that he understood as central mediators of the illness experience: automatic thoughts, schemata, and cognitive distortions. Automatic thoughts, often implicit and unrecognized, reflect themes of incompetence, defeat, hopelessness, deprivation, isolation, and guilt; his formulation of the "cognitive triad" encompasses the individual's negative thoughts about oneself, the world, and the future. Beck assumed that automatic thoughts reflect the person's overly negative interpretation of circumstances rather than a realistic appraisal of actual conditions, perpetuating maladaptive emotional and behavioral reactions.

Mental structures or schemata, made up of deep, tacit assumptions, beliefs, formulas, and rules that operate outside the usual range of awareness, guide the ways in which we perceive situations and process information (Beck, 1979; Beck & Dozios, 2011; Wakefield & Baer, 2010). Following Piaget's formulations, Beck assumes that we are predisposed to assimilate experience along the lines of existing schemata rather than to accommodate our cognitive structures to reflect discrepant or unexpected events. In developing his "cognitive specificity hypothesis," Beck proposes that patterns of thinking and themes of threat or loss vary across conceptions of psychopathology.

He describes representative types of errors in processing experience believed to underlie cognitive distortion, including dichotomous thinking (categorizing experience in absolute terms); arbitrary inferences (drawing negative conclusions without supporting evidence); selective abstraction (focusing on negative aspects of a situation and failing to consider positive elements); overgeneralization (developing fixed beliefs on the basis of a single incident and applying them across situations); and personalization (relating external events to oneself).

Beck emphasizes the process of "collaborative empiricism" in his conceptions of the therapeutic relationship. The patient and the clinician clarify focal concerns, establish goals, and explore connections between thoughts, feelings, actions, and events, working to identify "distorted" or "faulty" cognitions. Patients document negative patterns of thinking in a systematic fashion. The therapist and patient engage in Socratic dialogue, challenging beliefs and testing hypotheses through experiential learning, and forming alternative interpretations on the basis of evidence (Leahy, 2008).

In accord with Dewey's emphasis on experiential learning, Beck emphasizes the role of empiricism—learning by doing—in the process of change, encouraging patients to regard beliefs as hypotheses to be tested through "behavioral experiments" and reflections on experience. The patient and therapist develop tasks and activities to help them test beliefs and experiment with different behaviors in life situations. Behavioral approaches outlined in the preceding chapter, including methods of activation, problem-solving, rehearsal, social skills training, exposure, and relaxation procedures, help patients revise maladaptive beliefs and automatic thoughts as they generate experience and evidence that disconfirm current schemata. For Beck, cognitive change is a prerequisite to enduring change in emotion and behavior.

Constructivist Model: Meichenbaum

Although Donald Meichenbaum developed his original formulations of cognitive-behavior therapy in accordance with the basic assumptions of the rationalist perspective that had shaped the models of Ellis and Beck, he came to embrace the constructivist point of view as he expanded his conceptions of therapeutic action, bridging narrative perspectives and methods of intervention developed in the behavioral and cognitive paradigms. Drawing on a range of intellectual traditions, encompassing the philosophical writings of Kant, Wundt, and Cassirer; the cognitive research of Vygotsky, Piaget, and Kelly; narrative psychology; and the existential perspective of Frankl, he assumes that we create personal worlds of meaning. There are "multiple realities," and the task of psychotherapy is to help us realize the ways in which ongoing accounts of our experience perpetuate particular ways of feeling, thinking, and acting.

Following Bruner, he proposes that we are natural storytellers, representing ourselves and our realities in the form of narratives. The metaphor of the "constructive narrative" guides his conceptions of therapeutic action. We construct stories to account for our symptoms and problems in living, and he thinks of the therapist as a co-creator, joining the patient in reformulations of personal narratives and life stories. The practitioner functions as an empathic listener, following the patient's accounts of experience and collaborating in efforts to create more adaptive and functional renderings of past events, current circumstances, and the anticipated future.

His methods encompass reflective listening, focused exploration and reconstruction of traumatic events, Socratic questioning, in-vivo activities that sponsor experiential learning, and structured tasks that foster the development of problem-solving and coping skills. Like third-wave behavior therapists, Meichenbaum emphasizes the crucial importance of attunement, empathy, acceptance, and validation in establishing the therapeutic alliance, and the role of emotion in processing experience and creating meaning.

He believes that it is not the symptoms of stress, trauma, depression or anxiety per se that compromise functioning; instead, he proposes, what we say to ourselves and to others about our reactions and the stories we construct about our experience influence patterns of coping and adaptation.

The patient and therapist process the experience of suffering and challenge, collaborating in efforts to formulate a "'healing theory' of what happened and why" (Meichenbaum, 1995, p. 150). The task is to help patients "construct narratives that fit their present circumstances, that are coherent, and that prove plausible in capturing and explaining their difficulties" (1995, p. 150). In working from a narrative perspective, patients reformulate life experience in ways that deepen their understanding of the origins and meanings of current problems in living, and, as Roy Schafer emphasizes, "do so in a way that makes change conceivable and attainable" (1980, p. 38).

Realizing the crucial role of personal agency, self-efficacy, and mastery in the dynamics of change and growth, Meichenbaum challenges patients to summon examples of their capacities and strengths as they elaborate new ways of seeing themselves and their world, strengthening a sense of hope and possibility. He draws on a range of cognitive and behavioral methods in efforts to foster the development of problem-solving skills and coping strategies through various forms of experiential learning (see Meichenbaum, 2017, for an expanded review of his therapeutic approach, bridging narrative perspectives and cognitive-behavioral methods of intervention).

Integrative Model: Berlin

In her critiques of cognitive therapy, Sharon Berlin observed that thinkers locate the origins of what is the matter largely within the person, emphasizing the constructed features of personal meaning but failing to take account of the concrete particularity of actual circumstances in the social surround that perpetuate vulnerability and problems in functioning. Many of our most vulnerable patients must negotiate ongoing threat, adversity, deprivation, and trauma, she reasoned, and we cannot reduce their suffering and problems in living to "faculty beliefs," "cognitive distortions" or "irrational thoughts."

Berlin set out to expand the scope of the cognitive paradigm, introducing an integrative perspective that would challenge practitioners to take more account of the ways in which social and cultural conditions influence problems in living (Berlin, 2002, 2010). She drew on developments in neuroscience, personality and social psychology, relational psychoanalysis, experiential psychotherapy, narrative studies, and the framing perspectives of the social work tradition in fashioning her approach, focusing on the ways in which we use information to create meaning.

She assumes that we work continually to make sense of day to day life, and the meanings we elaborate—ongoing views of self, others, past events, and anticipated future—are shaped largely by two factors: first, the nature of the information we encounter in our readings of inner experience, relational life, and the social surround; and second, the schemata or memory patterns that guide our particular ways of processing events.

As a social worker she is particularly concerned with the ways in which depriving and oppressive conditions perpetuate problems in living and restrictions of opportunity. The therapeutic process centers on sources of information and schemata, seeking to help patients develop more functional ways of processing experience, creating meaning, and negotiating problems in living.

Drawing on basic principles of change formulated in cognitive psychology, she assumes that we change our minds only when we encounter circumstances or realize personal capacities that are different from what we have known. It is crucial, accordingly, to create discrepancies which challenge existing schemata and bring about new options and opportunities.

In her conceptions of change she emphasizes the crucial functions of stability and difference, drawing on Piagetian formulations of assimilation and accommodation. We must recognize difference in order to change, Berlin realizes, but the potential for growth is counterbalanced by our need to preserve coherence in sense of self and continuity in life experience. We are more likely to recognize and make use of difference when we are able to maintain stability. To be useful, accordingly, new information must be recognizable to existing memory patterns but different enough to bring about a meaningful shift.

She distinguishes two levels of change in her model, the first centered on sources of information, the second focused on schemata or memory systems. If problematic meanings originate in limited knowledge, the clinician seeks to help the patient generate new sources of information and integrate them into current schemata. New cues activate and strengthen adaptive patterns of functioning. In the second level of change, the clinician focuses on rigid, restrictive schemata that perpetuate problems in functioning, trying to help patients recognize preexisting patterns and make use of new information in the reorganization of schemata and development of new memory systems.

The task of intervention, broadly understood, is to identify and redress the contributions of sources of information and reorganize rigid, limited schemata that perpetuate problems in living. In her formulations of change and growth, Berlin emphasizes the role of action in efforts to create more positive meanings and strengthen memory patterns for mastery and possibility. Drawing on traditional behavioral approaches, she outlines strategies that help to bring about change, including instruction, modeling, skills training, and methods of exposure. Although the therapeutic process focuses on circumscribed problems in functioning, the more fundamental goal is to strengthen capacities and skills to engage in effective action—learning by doing, in Dewey's phrase—fostering the experience of personal agency, competence, and mastery.

Therapeutic Action

The orienting perspectives of the cognitive paradigm offer cogent accounts of therapeutic action as clinicians and patients formulate their understanding of what is the matter and what carries the potential to help, focusing our attention on mental structures, beliefs and attitudes, the ways we create meaning, and patterns of thinking. As we have seen, two fundamental perspectives have shaped conceptions of intervention in the cognitive tradition, broadly characterized as "rationalist" and "constructivist." In accord with the divergent philosophical foundations underlying each perspective, thinkers differ in their beliefs about the nature of reality, the character of subjective experience, the functions of reason and emotion, and the dynamics of therapeutic action thought to sponsor change and growth (for expanded discussion see Arnkoff & Glass, 1992; Mahoney, 2003; Mahoney & Granvold, 2005; Wachtel, 1997, 2011).

From the perspective of the rationalist approach, we come to know an outer world of reality through experience and cognition. Presumably, logical reasoning and explicit beliefs govern the dynamics of emotion and behavior. A range of problems in living originate in irrational, distorted patterns of thinking that can be "corrected" through reason and logic. The task of psychotherapy, accordingly, is to help the patient clarify cognitive distortions, challenge faulty beliefs, and develop more rational, functional ways of thinking that take account of actual circumstances and realistic prospects. The clinician serves as the arbiter of reality and rationality, attempting to clarify inaccurate assumptions, distortions, and errors in thinking in accord with what we take to be a consensual reality. The therapist challenges maladaptive thoughts, generating sources of experiential learning and evidence that help us test hypotheses, develop rational and realistic ways of understanding circumstances, expand coping capacities, and strengthen skills. Emotion is treated largely as a reflection of dysfunction or as an epiphenomenon (see Kazdin, 2008).

Constructivist approaches, influenced by the interpretive perspectives of postmodern thought and narrative psychology, assume that our experience of reality is mediated by subjectivity. In accord with developments in affective neuroscience and interpersonal neurobiology, thinkers understand emotion as a core constituent of the self, creating the subjective experience of being alive, serving as a fundamental mode of knowing, instrumental in the creation of meaning. Although the outer world places limits on the viability of the meanings we create, reality is not fixed or "out there" to be found; rather, we construct our experience of the world in particular linguistic, social, and cultural surrounds, and we regard the meanings we create as ongoing, contingent ways of making sense of events. We do not have access to a reality beyond our cognitive constructions.

From this perspective, the therapeutic process challenges us to explore the functional outcomes of our ways of seeing and understanding, focusing not on the truth or falsity of our accounts but on the practical outcomes of our thoughts that influence states of self, problem-solving, coping, and growth. In this sense constructivist approaches converge with the pragmatic philosophy of William James, emphasizing the practical outcomes of our thoughts. The clinician and patient explore the origins and development of beliefs and assumptions, patterns of thinking, and narrative accounts, considering their strength, coherence, and viability, co-creating formulations of experience that deepen meaning and sponsor growth.

The rationalist and constructivist perspectives continue to influence understanding and practice across the cognitive paradigm. In more pure versions of the rationalist approach, as discussed, we think of cognition as *the* causal mechanism of dysfunction, assuming that cognitive processes precipitate maladaptive patterns of emotion and behavior through selective perception, memory, and recall, activating vicious circles of thought, feeling, and action. Although traditional models continue to emphasize the role of cognition in dysfunction, change and growth, clinical scholars increasingly consider the dynamics of interoceptive experience, emotion, meaning, and context in reformulating conceptions of therapeutic action, rejecting the unidirectional models of causality that Ellis and Beck had proposed in their original approaches, recognizing the complexity and interdependence of biological, psychological, and social processes believed to govern the dynamics of thought, feeling, and action.

We can understand thoughts both as causes and as effects of sensation, emotion, and behavior, as constructivist thinkers had argued, introducing complex systems models of functioning. The ways in which we think about matters can influence how we feel and what we do, as Ellis and Beck believed. But the experience of sensation, feeling, imagery, and action, as well as the concrete particulars of our surrounds and circumstances, also activate schemata and shape ways of thinking. As Paul Wachtel observes:

> There is *always* some basis in reality for our experience. *And* there is always a significant contribution that reflects the active, constructive nature of all perceptual processes. Our thoughts, our perception, our association, our actions, are always a joint product of "internal" and "external" influences and processes.
>
> (2011, p. 110)

Over the last quarter century cognitive neuroscientists have documented the dynamics of unconscious processes in experimental research, as discussed in earlier chapters, and empirical findings show that implicit associative networks influence motivations, thoughts, feelings, and actions out of awareness. Even so, cognitive formulations of therapeutic action continue to center largely on conscious, explicit patterns of thought, feeling, and behavior, engaging the functions of the left brain. In working from a traditional cognitive model, clinical scholars have cautioned, therapists may overvalue conscious thought, reason, and language, privileging the functions of the left hemisphere, failing to attend to the more complex dynamics of sensation, emotion, and imagery mediated by the unconscious processes of the right hemisphere.

"Whatever elements an act of cognition may imply," William James had proposed, "it at least implies the existence of a feeling" (1909/1978, p. 179). Following developments in the field of affective neuroscience, we have deepened our understanding of the ways in which emotion organizes and integrates biological, psychological, and social domains of experience, linking mental processes over time, regulating states of self (Damasio, 2018; Siegel, 2020). Researchers distinguish "self-control" modes of emotional regulation that engage the executive functions of the left hemisphere—attempting to help us change the way we feel by consciously changing the way we think—from core regulatory processes mediated by the right hemisphere, believed to play a more fundamental role in modulating states of self and adaptive functioning (Greenberg, 2007, 2008, 2014; Schore, 2019a, 2019b).

In light of these different domains of function and modes of regulation, clinical scholars emphasize the need to expand traditional models of cognitive therapy, integrating relational and experiential approaches that foster the exploration, formulation, and validation of emotion in contrast to classical versions of intervention that focus on conscious attempts to control or change feelings, often treated as signs of dysfunction or as epiphenomena.

While rationalist versions of cognitive intervention continue to emphasize notions of challenge in formulations of therapeutic action, a growing number of practitioners have come to think of acceptance as a fundamental condition of change and growth, converging with developments in relational psychoanalysis, third-wave behavioral therapies, and humanistic approaches (see Chapters 5, 6, and 8). The therapist does not challenge the "irrational" or "unrealistic" features of beliefs or thoughts, as noted in earlier discussion; rather, the clinician explores the ways in which the patient has come to make sense of experience, taking an accepting, validating approach. Practitioners reason that an accepting view of the patient's experience can in itself alter patterns of thought and ways of seeing the self that perpetuate problems in living, strengthening engagement in activities that foster the development of capacities and skills instrumental in regulation of emotion and coping. Recent research has documented the critical role of acceptance as a fundamental mechanism of regulation in mindfulness interventions, emphasizing the need to provide training in attention monitoring skills and acceptance skills (Lindsay & Cresswell, 2019).

Neuroscience and Therapeutic Action

Empirical lines of study in the science of mind emphasize the fundamental role of neural integration in the organization of the self, emotional regulation, and functional behavior, as described in Part II. Reviews of research in the field of interpersonal neurobiology show that a range of symptoms and patterns of behavior encompassed in our conceptions of psychopathology are correlated with dysregulation and compromise of metabolic function in the cortical and subcortical regions of the brain (Cozolino, 2017; Kandel, 2018; LeDoux, 2015; Sapolsky, 2017; Schore, 2019a, 2019b; Siegel, 2020).

By way of example, symptoms of depression are associated with lower levels of metabolism in the left region of the prefrontal cortex and higher levels of activation in the right region of the prefrontal cortex. States of arousal and flashbacks following onset of post-traumatic stress disorder are correlated with higher levels of activation in the limbic region and the medial frontal structures of the right hemisphere; emotional arousal is also associated with decreased metabolism in the expressive language regions of the left hemisphere, compromising the ability to formulate and process experience (see case report of Jonathan in Chapter 9). Symptoms of obsessive-compulsive disorder are linked with activation of the middle sections of the frontal cortex and a subcortical structure known as the caudate nucleus (see Cozolino, 2017; Kandel, 2018;

Sapolsky, 2017; and Siegel, 2020 for expanded review and discussion of empirical findings).

On the basis of our current understanding of brain function, clinical scholars assume that cortical processing of sensations, feelings, thoughts, and behavior associated with a range of problems in functioning fosters the integration of neural networks through the activation of top-down mechanisms, strengthening capacities for emotional regulation and functional behavior. Presumably, the engagement of cortical functions through the conscious formulation and processing of subjective experience and behavior enhances activity in the left hemisphere and modulates right hemispheric and subcortical activation, strengthening vertical and horizontal domains of regulation and integration.

Exploration of the neurobiological correlates of psychotherapy has focused largely on traditional versions of cognitive-behavioral therapy, the most actively researched form of intervention, emphasized in evidence-based practice. Employing a range of brain imaging techniques, including the functional neuroimaging technologies of positron emission tomography and functional magnetic resonance imaging, researchers have documented changes in brain structure and function following courses of cognitive behavioral therapy for a range of conditions, including unipolar depression, anxiety disorders, panic disorder, social phobia, eating disorders, obsessive-compulsive disorder, schizophrenia, and traumatic brain injury.

Although a full review of the empirical literature is beyond the scope of this discussion, work to date suggests that changes in brain activation parallel improvements in functioning (see Cozolino, 2017, for summary and discussion of empirical findings, detailing therapeutic outcomes and changes in domains of neural activation). Overall, findings show decreased activity in the limbic system, particularly in the amygdala, the orbitomedial region, and cingulate cortex, and increased activity in the dorsolateral prefrontal cortex—the "rational mind"—following courses of treatment (Collerton, 2013; LeDoux, 2015; Sapolsky, 2017). The outcomes of cognitive behavior therapy are correlated with decreased emotionality, reflected in reduced limbic activity, and enhanced capacities for reflection and thoughtfulness, associated with increased activity in the dorsolateral frontal region, supporting proposals that the therapeutic process reinstates the integrative functions of neural networks thought to regulate mood and activity.

Even so, it remains unclear to what extent patients maintain therapeutic gains over time. As noted in Chapters 3 and 4, meta-analyses of outcome studies suggest that the benefits of traditional forms of cognitive therapy and cognitive-behavioral intervention tend to decay following the end of treatment, whereas patients in psychodynamically oriented forms of therapy not only show gains but continue to improve following the course of treatment (see Shedler, 2010, for review of comparative studies). As discussed earlier, it is possible that more pure versions of cognitive behavioral therapy alter explicit forms of thought and action but fail to engage implicit domains of sensation and emotion and reorganize underlying neural networks that perpetuate vicious circles of thinking, feeling, and acting. Converging lines of study in the fields of neuroscience reaffirm the importance of engaging the dynamics of sensation, emotion, imagery, cognition, and behavior in the "working through" process, described most fully in psychodynamic accounts of therapeutic action (see Chapter 4).

Researchers assume that moderate arousal or "optimal stress" fosters neuroplasticity, learning, change, and growth, as noted in earlier in earlier discussion. A range of methods and activities encompassed in cognitive models of treatment potentially intensity the experience of emotion, challenging patients to reconsider assumptions, beliefs, and patterns of thought through various forms of activity and experiential learning. Most therapists integrate behavioral methods likely to intensify the experience of emotion, challenging patients to engage sensations, feelings, and thoughts associated with fear, avoidance, and problems in living.

Drawing on recent developments in interpersonal neurobiology and attachment studies, clinical scholars assume that the therapeutic relationship and the interactive experience of help and care potentially activate bonding processes associated with neuroplasticity, strengthening capacities to regulate emotion, engage relational life, and initiate activities that sponsor change and growth. Beck had assumed that the core conditions of the therapeutic relationship would facilitate efforts to establish a "collaborative empiricism" and carry out the tasks and activities of intervention, creating opportunities to learn from experience, bringing about cognitive and symptomatic change. Although the earliest models of cognitive therapy emphasized technical procedures rather than the role of the therapeutic relationship, paralleling classical models of intervention in the behavioral paradigm, practitioners have increasingly recognized the role of the therapeutic alliance, acceptance, validation, collaboration, and the dynamics of interactive experience in reformulating conceptions of change and growth (see Castonguay, Constantino, McAleavy & Goldfried, 2011; Cattie, Buchholz & Abramowitz, 2020).

Researchers propose that the dynamics of interactive experience and the co-creation of narrative accounts and elaboration of life stories over the course of the therapeutic process engage the functions of the left and right hemispheres, fostering neural integration. As noted in Chapter 2, the autonoetic, analogical, context-dependent, mentalizing functions of the right hemisphere shape the imagery and themes of the narrative process, while the left hemisphere mediates interpretive and linguistic processing of content (Siegel, 2020). Constructivist perspectives, as we have seen, emphasize the role of meaning in functional outcomes as patients and therapists reformulate accounts of events and elaborate personal narratives that sponsor change and growth (for review of process-oriented models, see Hayes & Hoffman, 2018).

Concluding Comments

As we have seen, the earliest versions of cognitive therapy emerged from a rationalist epistemology, emphasizing technical methods and sources of experiential learning intended to help patients develop functional patterns of thought believed to govern emotion and behavior in accord with a consensual reality. Over time clinical scholars expanded the scope of treatment, introducing constructivist and relational perspectives, emphasizing the role of emotion, acceptance, validation, interactive experience, narrative, meaning, and context in change and growth. Researchers have documented the efficacy and effectiveness of cognitive approaches for a range of disorders and problems in functioning, and they are actively promoted as empirically supported forms of treatment, shaping models of evidence-based practice.

As in the behavioral paradigm, some cognitively oriented clinicians in the evidence-based practice movement continue to embrace nomothetic models of intervention based on a technical rationality, relying on standardized protocols for the treatment of specific symptoms associated with particular diagnostic classifications. From the perspective of clinical pragmatism, however, we recognize the crucial role of the therapeutic relationship, collaboration, co-creation of narrative and meaning, and various kinds of experiential learning in flexible, idiographic approaches to therapy. We potentially combine ideas and methods from a range of models as we carry out "experiments in adapting to need," searching for what proves useful in the particular circumstances of the clinical situation. As in the behavioral paradigm, basic concepts and methods lend themselves to applications in integrative approaches across the foundational schools of thought.

References

Arnkoff, D. & Glass, C. R. (1992). Cognitive therapy and psychotherapy integration, in D. K. Freedheim (Ed.), *History of psychotherapy: A century of change* (pp. 657–694). Washington, DC: American Psychological Association.

Batchelor, S. (2017). *Secular Buddhism*. New Haven, CT: Yale University Press.

Beck, A. (Ed.) (1979). *Cognitive therapy of depression*. New York: Guilford.

Beck, A. & Dozois, D. J. (2011). Cognitive therapy: Current status and future directions. *Annual Review of Medicine*, 62, 397–409.

Berlin, S. (2002). *Clinical social work: A cognitive-integrative approach*. New York: Oxford University Press.

Berlin, S. (2010). Why cognitive therapy needs social work, in W. Borden (Ed.), *Reshaping theory in contemporary social work* (pp. 31–51). New York: Columbia University Press.

Borden, W. (2010). Taking multiplicity seriously: Pluralism, pragmatism, and integrative perspectives in clinical social work, in W. Borden (Ed.), *Reshaping theory in contemporary social work* (pp. 3–31). New York: Columbia University Press.

Bruner, J. (1990). *Acts of meaning*. Cambridge, MA: Harvard University Press.

Castonguay, L., Constantino, M., McAleavey, A. & Goldfried, M. (2011). The therapeutic alliance in cognitive behavioral therapy, in C. Muran & J. P. Barber (Eds.). *The therapeutic alliance: An evidence-based guide to practice* (pp. 150–171). New York: Guilford.

Cattie, J., Buchholz, J. & Abramowitz, J. (2020). Cognitive therapy and cognitive-behavioral therapy, in S. Messer & N. Kaslow (Eds.), *Essential psychotherapies*, (pp. 142–182). New York: Guilford.

Collerton, J. (2013). Psychotherapy and brain plasticity. *Frontiers in psychology*, 4, 548.

Cozolino, L. (2017). *The neuroscience of psychotherapy*, 3rd edn. New York: Norton.

Damasio, A. (2018). *The strange order of things: Life, feeling, and the making of cultures.* New York: Vintage.

DeRubeis, R. J., Keefe, J. R. & Beck, A. T. (2019). Cognitive therapy, in S. Dobson & D. Dozois (Eds.), *Handbook of cognitive-behavioral therapy* (pp. 218–248). New York: Guilford.

Dowd, T. & McClearly, A. (2007). Elements of Buddhist philosophy in cognitive psychotherapy, *Journal of Cognitive and Behavioural psychotherapies*, 7, 67–79.

Ellenberger, H. (1970). *The discovery of the unconscious.* New York: Basic Books.

Ellis, A. (1962). *Reason and emotion in psychotherapy.* New York: Lyle Stuart.

Ellis, A. & Bernard, M. (Eds.) (1985). *Clinical applications of rational emotive therapy.* New York: Plenum Press.

Epstein, M. (2018). *Advice not given: A guide to getting over yourself.* New York: Penguin.

Erdelyi, M. (1985). *Psychoanalysis: Freud's cognitive psychology.* New York: W. H. Freeman.

Greenberg, L. (2007). Emotion coming of age. *Clinical Psychology Science and Practice*, 14, 414–421.

Greenberg, L. (2008). Emotion and cognition in psychotherapy: The transforming power of affect. *Canadian Psychology*, 49 (1), 49–59.

Greenberg, L. (2014). The therapeutic relationship in emotion-focused therapy. *Psychotherapy*, 51, 350–357.

Gyatso, T. (2005). *The universe in a single atom.* New York: Morgan Road Books.

Hayes, S. & Hoffman, S. G. (2018). *Process-based CBT: The science and core competencies of cognitive behavioral therapy.* Oakland, CA: New Harbinger.

James, W. (1909/1978). *Pragmatism and the meaning of truth.* Cambridge, MA: Harvard University Press.

Kabat-Zinn, J. (2013). *Full catastrophe living: Using the wisdom of your body and mind to face stress, pain, and illness.* New York: Bantam.

Kandel, E. (2012). *The age of insight.* New York: Farrar, Straus & Giroux.

Kandel, E. (2018). *The disordered mind.* New York: Farrar, Straus & Giroux.

Kazdin, A. (2008). Evidence-based treatment and practice. *American Psychologist*, 63 (3), 146–159.

Lazarus, R. & Folkman, S. (1984). *Stress, appraisal, and coping.* New York: Springer.

Leahy, R. L. (2008). The therapeutic relationship in cognitive-behavioral therapy. *Behavioural and Cognitive Psychotherapy*, 36 (6), 769–777.

LeDoux, J. (2015). *Anxiety.* New York: Viking.

Lindsay, E. K. & Cresswell, J. D. (2019). Mechanisms of mindfulness training: Monitor and acceptance theory. *Clinical Psychology Review*, 51, 48–59.

Mahoney, M. (1995). *Cognitive and constructive therapies: Theory, research, and practice.* New York: Springer.

Mahoney, M. (2003). *Constructive psychotherapy: A practical guide.* New York: Guilford.

Mahoney, M. (2004). Synthesis, in A. Freeman, M. J. Mahoney, P. Devito & D. Martin (Eds.), *Cognition and psychotherapy.* New York: Springer.

Mahoney, M. & Granvold, D. (2005). Constructivism and psychotherapy. *World Psychiatry*, 4 (2), 74–77.

Meichenbaum, D. (1995). Cognitive-behavioral therapy in historical perspective, in B. Bognar & L. Beutler (Eds.), *Comprehensive textbook of psychotherapy*. New York: Oxford.

Meichenbaum, D. (2017). *The evolution of cognitive behavior therapy*. New York: Routledge.

Messer, S. & Wachtel, P. (1997). Theoretical perspectives in psychotherapy, in D. Freedheim (Ed.), *History of psychotherapy* (pp. 105–107). Washington, DC: American Psychological Association.

Neimeyer, R. (2009). *Constructivist psychotherapy*. New York: Routledge.

Safran, J. (1998). *Widening the scope of cognitive therapy*. Northvale, NJ: Jason Aronson.

Sapolsky, R. (2017). *Behave*. New York: Penguin.

Schafer, R. (1980). Narration in the psychoanalytic dialogue. *Critical Inquiry*, 7, 29–53.

Schore, A. (2019a) *The development of the unconscious mind*. New York: Norton.

Schore, A. (2019b). *Right brain psychotherapy*. New York: Norton.

Segal, Z. V., Williams, M. & Teasdale, J. D. (2013). *Mindfulness-based cognitive therapy for depression*, 2nd edn. New York: Guilford.

Shedler, J. (2010). The efficacy of psychodynamic psychotherapy. *American Psychologist*, 65 (2), 98–109.

Siegel, D. (2020). *The developing mind*, 3rd edn. New York: Guilford.

Wachtel, P. (1997). *Psychoanalysis, behavior therapy, and the outside world*. New York: Guilford.

Wachtel, P. (2008). *Relational theory and the practice of psychotherapy*. New York: Guilford.

Wachtel, P. (2011). *Therapeutic communication*, 2nd edn. New York: Guilford

Wakefield, J. & Baer, J. (2010). The cognitivization of psychoanalysis: Toward an integration of psychodynamic and cognitive theories, in W. Borden (Ed.), *Reshaping theory in contemporary social work* (pp. 51–81). New York: Columbia University Press.

Westen, D. (2005). Implications of research in cognitive neuroscience for psychotherapy, in G. Gabbard, J. Beck & J. Holmes (Eds.), *Oxford textbook of psychotherapy* (pp. 443–448). New York: Oxford University Press.

Wright, L. (2017). *Why Buddhism is true*. New York: Simon & Schuster.

8   The Humanistic Paradigm

...in every individual there is a uniqueness that defies all formulation.

–William James

The humanistic paradigm emerged as the "Third Force" in American psychology after World War II as scholars and psychotherapists challenged reductive renderings of classical psychoanalysis and the mechanistic limits of behaviorism. A range of thinkers and intellectual traditions have shaped understanding and practice in the humanistic schools of thought over the last half century. Clinicians have drawn on phenomenological, existential, constructivist, and experiential perspectives in developing conceptions of personality, vulnerability, and therapeutic action, and recent theorizing has been shaped by developments in fields of affective neuroscience and interpersonal neurobiology. Practitioners have embraced fundamental concerns that converge with the principles and values of clinical pragmatism, emphasizing the individuality of the person and subjective experience; notions of agency, intention and will; exercise of freedom and choice; the crucial functions of the therapeutic relationship, collaboration, and dialogue; the co-creation of narrative and meaning; the dynamics of experiential learning, and inherent capacities for change, growth, and realization of potential in the individuation of the self. The field of psychotherapy research originated in the humanistic paradigm, shaped by the pioneering studies of Carl Rogers. Over the years researchers have demonstrated the efficacy and effectiveness of person-centered and experiential approaches, documenting the crucial role of the therapeutic relationship in outcomes.

In this chapter I review the emergence of the humanistic paradigm, outlining orienting perspectives and fundamental concerns, and explore the ways in which concepts of therapeutic action deepen our understanding of core processes believed to bring about change and growth. As in the preceding chapters, I begin with a brief account of the intellectual traditions that have shaped the development of the paradigm and trace the evolution of clinical practice. I outline three models that exemplify the defining features of the paradigm, focusing on the person-centered approach of Carl Rogers and experiential approaches introduced by Eugene Gendlin and Leslie Greenberg.

In doing so I consider the ways in which recent developments in the science of mind and the principles and values of clinical pragmatism deepen our appreciation of essential concerns in our understanding of therapeutic action, change, and growth.

Origins

A range of intellectual traditions in philosophy and psychology have shaped the development of humanistic thought and values in contemporary psychotherapy. Historians trace the origins of the humanist tradition to Socrates and Plato, who rejected materialism as a means of understanding human experience, distinguishing the psyche or soul from the physical body. We are living beings—souls, selves—subjects, not objects, experiencing, feeling, thinking, willing, and acting. The Aristotelian notion of the observer studying the person as an object fails to capture the essence of what it means to be human.

Humanistic perspectives emerged in the Renaissance as the authoritarian traditions of scholastic philosophy and theology that had shaped the assumptive world of the Middle Ages receded and scholars rediscovered the classical ideals of ancient Rome and Greece. They emphasized the dignity and worth of the person as an individual and the belief that reason, will, and action can foster the development of the individual and the common good, improving worldly conditions. The portraiture of Renaissance art captured the subjectivity and complexity of human individuality (Barzun, 2000).

A series of European philosophers introduced concerns and ideas in the 19th century that influenced existential and phenomenological conceptions of humanistic psychology and psychotherapy. Soren Kierkegaard emphasized the crucial role of experiential reflection, freedom, and responsibility in his accounts of consciousness, self, and cultural life (1844/1944). Friedrich Nietzsche distinguished "Apollonian" and "Dionysian" views of life in his vision of the human situation. In the deepest, fullest model of living, he proposes, we come to embrace the dialectical interplay between the divergent visions of reality and illusion, experiencing "the whole range and wealth of being natural" (1889/1982, p. 554).

Edmund Husserl, Martin Heidegger, and Karl Jaspers elaborated phenomenological perspectives in the 20th century, arguing that we must take account of the subjectivity of the individual if we are to fully grasp the nature of human experience. The fundamental task of phenomenology, Husserl proposed, is to apprehend human experience in the subjective context of its living reality. Heidegger drew on the existential formulations of Kierkegaard and the phenomenological methods of Husserl, his mentor, in fashioning a philosophy of being. He challenged the Western tradition that had made clear distinctions between "inner experience" and "outer realities" in his notion of "being-in-the-world," arguing that we cannot separate the "subjective" and the "objective" from the standpoint of experience (Heidegger, 1962; Husserl, 1913/1962).

William James believed that the individual carries a "uniqueness that defies all formulation," as noted in the account of clinical pragmatism in Chapter 1 (James, 1911/1979, p. 109). He rejected mechanistic accounts of mental life, as we saw in our discussion of the mind-body problem in Chapter 2, arguing that psychology should focus on the whole person: "The only states of consciousness that we naturally deal with are found in personal consciousnesses, minds, selves, concrete particular I's and you's" (1890, p. 497). His conception of "the stream of consciousness" follows from his deep appreciation of subjectivity. More than anything, he emphasizes, our experience is *personal*: Every sensation, feeling, image, thought, or action is mine, or hers, or his, or yours: "The universal conscious fact is not 'feelings and thoughts exist,' but 'I think' and 'I feel.' No psychology… can question the existence of personal selves" (1890, p. 499).

Evolution of Therapeutic Practice

As we have seen, the determinism of Freud's drive psychology moved a series of thinkers to establish humanistic perspectives in the broader psychodynamic paradigm, as outlined in Chapters 4 and 5. Carl Jung, Alfred Adler, and Otto Rank, originally members of Freud's inner circle, challenged his biological perspective and elaborated independent schools of thought that emphasized subjectivity and personal meaning, existential concerns, and the role of relationship, social life, and culture in development, health, and well-being.

Jung described the ways in which emerging concerns, values, and organizing purposes shape efforts to realize potential and work toward the individuation of the self in adulthood and later life. Adler introduced a psychology of values that emphasized subjectivity and personal meaning; notions of will, self-determination, and responsibility; creativity and capacities for transcendence; and the crucial role of relational life and social surrounds in health, well-being, and the common good. Rank, like Adler, centered on concepts of will, self-determination, and responsibility in elaborating his developmental formulations and existential perspective.

Donald Winnicott proposed that we are born with an inherent drive to actualize the "true self," the inviolate core of our being, and described the "maturational process" that governs the development of the individual. He introduced a language of subjectivity in his efforts to represent core states of self, exploring the experience of aliveness, authenticity, creativity, wonder, and play in everyday life. Like Winnicott, Karen Horney understood our tendency to actualize the "real" self as a cardinal motivation in human development. She described neurosis as "a special form of development antithetical to growth" (1950, p. 13), reaffirming her belief in our fundamental "wish to grow and to leave nothing untouched that prevents growth" (1942, p. 175, cited in Rogers, 1951/1965, p. 489).

Existential perspectives emerged in Europe as thinkers attempted to come to terms with the sense of alienation and vulnerability that followed the two

World Wars. Drawing on the philosophical thought of Kierkegaard, Nietzsche, Husserl, Jaspers, and Heidegger, thinkers challenged the biological perspective of Freud, rejecting his deterministic and mechanistic renderings of the human situation. They embraced notions of personal agency and will; freedom, choice, and responsibility; and the crucial role of guiding purposes as we work to create meaning and fulfill our desire to live.

Ludwig Binswanger and Medard Boss, trained as psychiatrists in Switzerland, created an approach based on Heidegger's notion of Dasein, known as Daseinanalyse (Binswanger, 1951/1963; Boss, 1957/1963). Working from a phenomenological perspective, they emphasized the need to enter the experiential world of the patient, exploring the ways in which we give meaning to existence.

Victor Frankl, practicing as a psychiatrist in Vienna, introduced logotherapy, an approach originating in his experience as a prisoner in the Nazi death camp at Auschwitz. He thought of the "will to meaning" as the cardinal motivation in human experience, realized in unique and particular ways by each individual over the course of life (1963). Rollo May, trained as a psychoanalyst at the William Alanson White Institute in New York, introduced the European existentialists to psychotherapists in the United States in a series of writings, beginning with his seminal work, *The meaning of anxiety* (May, 1950/1977). Irvin Yalom would expand conceptions of therapeutic action in his classic text, *Existential psychotherapy*, published in 1980.

Kurt Goldstein, working as a neurologist and psychiatrist in Germany after World War I, documented the ways in which soldiers constructed their world anew following traumatic brain injury, expanding capacities for coping and adaptation. He spoke of "the essence of the individual" and elaborated a holistic conception of the person, proposing that the experience of adversity and misfortune can sponsor growth and development in accord with our current understanding of neuroplasticity. He introduced the concept of the "self-actualizing tendency," a fundamental motivational force that mediates the course of development, guiding efforts to realize potential (Goldstein, 1934/1995, p. 162).

Frederick Perls, who had trained in neuropsychiatry in Berlin after serving in World War I, worked closely with Goldstein in his treatment of traumatic brain injury. He was influenced by Goldstein's holistic view of the individual and the "self-actualizing tendency" in forming his conceptions of gestalt therapy. He drew on a range of intellectual traditions as he continued to develop his clinical perspective, including phenomenological and existential thought; the gestalt psychology of K. Koffka, W. Kohler, and M. Wertheimer; the psychoanalytic contributions of Rank, Horney, and Wilhelm Reich; the field theory of Kurt Lewin; and fundamental elements of Zen. Over the course of his collaboration with Laura Perls, Paul Goodman, and Ralph Heferline, following his move to the United States in 1946, Perls deepened his exploration of concerns that would shape therapeutic practice in the broader humanistic paradigm, focusing on the domain of the body and interoceptive experience; the dynamics of sensation, feeling, thought, and behavior; awareness of the present moment; and authenticity and dialogue in the therapeutic relationship (Perls, 1947; Perls, Hefferline & Goodman, 1951).

In the domain of academic psychology a growing number of thinkers challenged the reductionism of Freudian thought and behaviorism that had failed to take account of fundamental aspects of human life. Gordon Allport, Henry Murray, Gardner Murphy, George Kelly, Carl Rogers, and Abraham Maslow expanded conceptions of personality, focusing on the unique experiential world of the individual, exploring conceptions of purpose, meaning, and realization of potential.

Maslow emerged as the principal architect of humanistic psychology in the 1950s, outlining fundamental concerns, themes, and assumptions that would shape understanding across the paradigm. He sought to establish what he thought of as a "Third Force" in psychology that would deal with matters of individuality, consciousness, values, ethics, purposes, and what he described as "'peak experience'—what you feel and perhaps 'know' when you gain authentic elevation as a human being" (Maslow, 1971, p. xvi; see also 1967a, 1968, 1970).

Like Jung, Winnicott, Horney, and Goldstein, Maslow believed that there is "an active will toward health, an impulse towards growth, or towards the actualization of human potentialities" (1967b, p. 153). In accord with Horney, he thought of neurosis as "a failure of personal growth," "a falling short of what one could have been, and even, one could say, of what one should have been, biologically speaking, that is, if one had grown and developed in an unimpeded way" (1971, p. 33). He provided case studies of historical and contemporary figures whom he regarded as exemplars of self-actualization and described the defining features of "peak experience" and "the higher reaches of human nature" found in the most fully developed individuals (1971, p. xvi).

Although Maslow did not set out to create a model of psychotherapy, his conceptual syntheses and empirical research would shape the assumptive world of clinical practice through the second half of the 20th century. Drawing on phenomenological and existential points of view, psychotherapists increasingly focused on the person as an individual, seeking to take account of capacities for reflective consciousness, agency and will, and purpose and meaning, emphasizing conceptions of growth that challenged reductive accounts of human experience in the psychoanalytic and behavioral paradigms.

Rogers emerged as a formative influence in the field of therapeutic practice over the course of his research and teaching in the 1950s and 1960s. He had created the first version of his approach, "non-directive therapy," in the 1940s, and he would emphasize the crucial role of acceptance, empathic understanding, and authenticity as he elaborated conceptions of the helping relationship and interactive experience, healing, and growth in the client-centered model.

Rogers drew on a range of thinkers in developing his conceptions of therapeutic action. He had begun doctoral study in ministry at Union Theological

Seminary in New York but left the program after two years to pursue training in clinical psychology at Columbia University, where one of his teachers, W. H. Kilpatrick, introduced him to the pragmatic philosophy of John Dewey. Like Maslow, he was influenced by Goldstein's holistic conception of the person and his formulations of the self-actualizing tendency. His training in psychodynamic psychotherapy deepened his appreciation of the humanistic orientations of Adler and Rank and the relational formulations of Horney and Harry Stack Sullivan. He worked as a psychologist in a child guidance clinic for 12 years before he began his academic career, teaching at Ohio State University, the University of Chicago, and the University of Wisconsin. He elaborated conceptions of personality; vulnerability and problems in living; health, well-being, and optimal functioning; and concepts of therapeutic action that would influence training and practice across the foundational schools of thought (see Rogers, 1942, 1951/1965, 1957, 1959, and 1961; see Kirschenbaum, 2009, for biographical account).

Clinical scholars continued to expand the scope of therapeutic action in the humanistic paradigm, introducing a range of experiential approaches that emphasized the realm of emotion, learning, and the active role of the clinician in helping patients challenge the dynamics of inner life that perpetuate problems in living. Eugene Gendlin, who had emigrated to the United States following the Nazi invasion of Vienna in 1938, received a doctoral degree in philosophy and began to collaborate with Rogers at the University of Chicago in 1953. He carried out research on therapeutic processes and outcomes and developed an experiential approach known as focusing, described in the following section.

Like Gendlin, Laura Rice worked closely with Rogers as a student at the University of Chicago in the 1950s and continued to carry out research on psychotherapy at York University in Toronto. She introduced a method known as task analysis, exploring core processes believed to facilitate change and growth over the course of therapy. She described a systematic, evocative unfolding procedure that outlines methods of engaging the processes of discovery and change (Rice, 1992). She collaborated with Leslie Greenberg, one of her graduate students, in developing an experiential approach known as emotion-focused therapy (Rice & Greenberg, 1984). Drawing on recent developments in affective neuroscience and interpersonal neurobiology, Greenberg and his collaborators have continued to elaborate a process-experiential approach to psychotherapy, building on classical Rogerian theory, integrating active methods from psychodynamic, cognitive, and behavioral schools of thought, described in the following section.

The person-centered perspective of Carl Rogers, experiential models, and existential approaches continue to influence formulations of therapeutic action in the wider humanistic paradigm (see Messer & Kaslow, 2020, for expanded reviews of person-centered, experiential, and existential schools of thought). More broadly, the orienting perspectives of humanistic psychotherapy have shaped practice across the foundational schools of thought, guiding the development of integrative approaches.

Models of Therapy

In this section I outline the defining features of Rogers' person-centered approach in greater detail and review experiential models developed by Eugene Gendlin and Leslie Greenberg and colleagues that exemplify overlapping conceptions of therapeutic action encompassed in the humanistic paradigm.

Person-Centered Approach: Rogers

Rogers assumes that the cardinal motivation in human development is to realize our potential and actualize the self. Building on Goldstein's formulation of the actualizing tendency, he proposes: "the organism has one basic tendency and striving—to actualize, maintain, and enhance the experiencing organism" (1951/1965, p. 487). In this sense he focuses on fundamental *processes* thought to foster change and growth, emphasizing the crucial importance of being present in the moment to make use of experiential opportunities in the realization of potential and the individuation of the self. We must be *open* to our experience of inner life and outer realities as we create more differentiated and integrated ways of being and living.

Rogers centers on the phenomenal field of the person in context, taking account of the concrete circumstances of particular situations in his conceptions of moment by moment functioning, realizing that our ongoing experience of relational life and social surrounds shapes what we feel, think, and do. In following the phenomenological perspective of Goldstein, he assumes that we do not live in a realm of objective reality but negotiate the world as we experience and construct it. We create our subjective sense of self and the world through experience, he believes, proposing that the internal frame of reference of the individual is the best vantage point for understanding feeling, thought, and action (1951/1965, p. 494).

Although Rogers recognizes the role of relational and contextual factors in his conceptions of development, he emphasizes the crucial role of personal agency, values, purposes, and meaning in his formulations of self-actualization, health, and well-being. In proposals that converge with Daniel Siegel's conceptions of development in interpersonal neurobiology, Rogers expanded his initial version of self-actualization to encompass what he imagines to be a broader organizing tendency operating in nature that moves all forms of life toward greater order, complexity, integration, and interrelatedness (Siegel, 2018, 2020).

We are born with an inherent capacity to value processes that we perceive as preserving or enhancing our lives, he proposes, just as we recognize experiences that threaten or limit our growth. Rogers anticipates formulations of "self-righting" processes described in conceptions of resilience (Bohart & Watson, 2020).

Our failure to function as a person in process, reflected in defensive, rigid, undifferentiated patterns of behavior, perpetuates vulnerability and problems in living. Rogers assumes that dysfunction follows from our failure to attend to the flow of experience in ways that facilitate problem-solving and coping. Presumably, feeling, thinking, and acting in ways that violate our most fundamental sense of self creates conflict, suffering, and demoralization, limiting the extent to which we can engage the actualizing tendency.

Rogers describes three domains of concern in his accounts of the fully functioning person: "openness to experience;" "existential living," reflected in spontaneous, flexible, functional ways of being and relating in moment by moment experience; and "organismic trusting" that shapes decision-making and behavior in light of needs, values, and essential concerns (Rogers, 1961, pp. 187–189). These concerns provide crucial points of reference over the course of the therapeutic process.

Rogers proposes that the fundamental dynamic of change in psychotherapy lies in our inherent capacities for growth and individuation; Arthur Bohart speaks of a "self-organizing wisdom" (Bohart & Watson, 2011, p. 246). The therapeutic process seeks to help the patient engage and strengthen capacities for self-actualization through the core conditions of the relationship and the interactive experience of exploration, reflection, support, and care.

Over the course of his research Rogers came to formulate the core conditions of the therapeutic relationship as unconditional positive regard, acceptance, and warmth; empathic understanding, reflected in the capacity to understand the subjective world of the patient; and genuineness or congruence, proposing that these characteristics are essential and often sufficient to bring about growth (Rogers, 1957, 1958a, 1958b). In the client-centered model of psychotherapy, the clinician's authenticity, attunement, empathic responsiveness, and acceptance of what the individual is experiencing facilitate efforts to explore inner states encompassing the domains of sensation, emotion, thought, and imagery.

Rogers describes the conditions of receptivity that operate in the experiential field and "psychological contact" between the therapist and the patient:

> The two people are to some degree in contact… each makes some perceived difference in the experiential field of the other. Probably it is sufficient if each member makes some "subceived" difference, even though the individual may not be consciously aware of this impact… it is almost certain that at some organic level he does sense this difference.
>
> (1957, p. 96)

The clinician follows the patient's lead in the sessions, focused on the moment by moment flow of sensation, feeling, imagery, and thought, engaging inherent capacities to guide the process of discovery and growth. The patient's experience of the therapist's presence and resonance, authenticity, acceptance and unconditional regard, and empathic immersion in experience fosters the process of change and growth.

Rogers assumes that the inherent strength of the actualizing tendency generates experience that leads to growth and fulfillment. The clinician works to clarify and convey understanding of the patient's experience through reflection of feeling and thought, clarifying the meaning of what has been related. In traditional Rogerian approaches, the clinician moves beyond explicit accounts of experience and explores what the patient is experiencing but not yet able to formulate. In following the classical client-centered approach, however, the therapist remains within the individual's current range in awareness of experience.

Although the therapeutic process carries the potential to deepen understanding and insight, Rogers rejects interpretive methods and believes that the core conditions of the relationship and the synchrony of interactive experience are the fundamental mechanisms of change and growth, helping patients strengthen capacities for processing the dynamics of inner life, negotiating problems in living, and actualizing the self. As we feel accepted, supported, and understood, Rogers believes, we are increasingly able to challenge defensive patterns of behavior, more fully experience emotion, express feelings, and develop capacities and skills in living through experiential learning.

Over the course of the therapeutic process, we negotiate incongruities between different feelings, thoughts, and actions and generate opportunities to strengthen and expand capacities and skills that foster new ways of being, relating, and living. Although person-centered therapists do not teach skills, they model ways of processing experience and provide occasions for observational learning. Patients work toward change in the *processes* of living, reflected in greater access to inner experience, acceptance of self, trust in the authority of subjective experience, values, and purposes; initiative in making decisions and acting on them; and capacities to assume responsibility for choices. The focus is on the whole person, rather than on symptoms or circumscribed problems, and the fundamental aim of psychotherapy is to help the individual strengthen capacities for authentic ways of being, relating, and living (for expanded accounts of classical and contemporary Rogerian approaches see Bohart & Watson, 2020).

Experiential Approaches

According to the principles of the classical Rogerian approach, as we have seen, we assume that the core conditions of the therapeutic relationship and the dynamics of interactive experience carry the potential to reinstate developmental processes, bringing about change and growth. The clinician takes a non-directive stance, accordingly, starting where the person is, believing that the therapeutic process will engage innate capacities for growth, realization of potential, and individuation of self through critical and creative intelligence (Bohart & Watson, 2020).

In expanding concepts of therapeutic action, practitioners have departed from the non-directive stance of the classical Rogerian approach, introducing active methods of intervention and guidance in efforts to help patients process emotions that perpetuate problems in living. The models of Gendlin and Greenberg and his collaborators exemplify the defining features of the experiential perspective.

Focusing: Gendlin

Over the course of his collaboration with Rogers, Gendlin created a theory of experiencing that served as the foundation for his method of focusing, an experiential approach that therapists have integrated in their practice across the foundational schools of thought. Although some clinicians think of focusing as a model of therapy, Gendlin describes it as a procedure that strengthens all forms of therapeutic practice (1991, 1996).

He assumes that our efforts to experience, formulate, and process bodily sensations and emotions create meaning, fostering change and growth (Gendlin, 1962, 1964). He conceives of experiencing as a fundamental way of knowing the dynamics of inner life and outer realities, describing it as the immediate, non-verbal sensing of patterns and relationships within the self and in the world. In light of our current understanding of brain structure and function we can think of experiencing as an implicit mode of processing information and knowing mediated largely by the right hemisphere of the brain, engaging "top-down" and "bottom-up" mechanisms of regulation.

Like Rogers, Gendlin believes that meaning generated through the embodied process of experiencing is more complex than the understanding we find through conscious, verbal, conceptual thought. In this sense he distinguishes "cognitive insight" from the experience of "emotional insight," as psychodynamic thinkers emphasize in their conceptions of the core processes believed to foster change and growth.

When we are fully functioning, Gendlin proposes, we engage the wider range of our faculties, thinking rationally as we draw on our experiential sense of what is meaningful and negotiate problems in living. If the flow of experiencing is disrupted, however, we are unable to process emotion and create meaning. In the absence of capacities to symbolize experience, we rely on fixed perceptions, beliefs, and attitudes—what he calls "frozen wholes"—that take the place of meaning. We are bound by mental structures, he proposes, and "the structures themselves are not modifiable by present occurrences" (1964, p. 129). He explains: "Instead of the many, many implicit meanings of experiencing which must interact with present detail to interpret and react, the individual has a structured feeling pattern" (1964, p. 129).

Gendlin thinks of focusing as a point of entry into a mode of sensing, and the aim of the procedure is to reinstate the process of experiencing. He emphasizes that practitioners must not engage "mental structures" but restore capacities for "functioning experience" (1964, p. 132). The therapist helps the individual attend to the "direct referents" or "felt sense" of concerns and explore their implicit meanings, modeling ways of processing subjective experience. In his account of the process he reflects: "Most people require certain special instructions to let a felt sense come. One has to place one's attention into the center of one's body, and sense what comes there in relation to some problem, situation, or aspect of life" (1991, p. 271). The "explication of felt meaning" symbolizes the experience in words, images, or gestures. The process seeks to bring about a "felt shift" that sponsors a fresh unfolding of meaning, releasing one from "frozen wholes," facilitating efforts to formulate experience and negotiate problems in functioning (for review of the structure and techniques of the procedure see Gendlin, 1996).

Gendlin centers our attention on the dynamics of bodily sensation, emotion, and meaning, strengthening experiential formulations of therapeutic action across the foundational schools of thought. He emphasizes the importance of exploring tacit information carried in bodily felt experience and the ways in which symbolization and expression of emotion fosters growth, well-being, and adaptive functioning.

Emotion-Focused Therapy: Greenberg

Greenberg observes that modern therapeutic approaches have privileged conscious understanding and cognitive and behavioral forms of change, failing to consider the domain of emotion. Drawing on recent developments in affective neuroscience and interpersonal neurobiology, Greenberg and his colleagues have expanded concepts of therapeutic action in the humanistic paradigm, continuing to elaborate what they describe as an integrative, experiential, process-oriented approach. In developing the model, they emphasize the central importance of the awareness, acceptance, and understanding of emotion; the visceral experience of emotion and bodily sensation in the therapeutic process; and the creation of meaning in change and growth (Greenberg, 2016).

Greenberg understands basic emotions—fear, anger, sadness, and disgust—as core constituents in the construction of complex frameworks that orient us to our environments. In his view, emotions are "purposive," shaping our motivations, perceptions, thoughts, and actions, playing a fundamental role in goal-directed behavior. He explains:

> Emotion sets a basic mode of processing in action. Fear sets in motion a fear processing mechanism that searches for danger, sadness informs us of loss, and anger informs us of violation. Emotions are also our primary system of communication... emotions determine much of who we are...
>
> (2016, p. 5)

He assumes that our capacities to process subjective experience and to recognize emotion as a mode of learning and knowing are fundamental in adaptive functioning, health, and well-being. Emotional competence or "emotional literacy" involves access to inner experience; the ability to regulate and transform maladaptive emotion; and the development of narratives that affirm sense of self and identity. He traces the origins of problems in living to four fundamental causes: lack of awareness, avoidance, or disavowal of emotion; dysregulation of emotion; maladaptive emotional responses; or difficulties in processing emotion and creating meaning that fosters coping, adaptation, and realization of potential. He emphasizes the role of emotion in change and growth, accordingly, believing that a range of problems in living originate in our failures to explore and engage the dynamics of inner life.

Greenberg distinguishes methods of therapeutic action that engage the executive functions of the left hemisphere, emphasized in cognitive and cognitive-behavioral models of intervention focused on conscious control of feelings, from experiential approaches believed to engage the mechanisms of the right hemisphere, instrumental in the regulation of unconscious, bodily based emotion. In following the process-oriented approach that he and his colleagues have developed, we do not attempt to help patients "change the way they feel by changing the way they think," but rather seek to help them embody, tolerate, and accept what they are feeling as they process experience, engaging the regulatory functions of the right hemisphere (Greenberg, 2007, p. 415). In accordance with developments in interpersonal neurobiology, reviewed in Chapter 2, Greenberg acknowledges that the "building up of implicit or automatic emotion regulation capacities" is a prerequisite of enduring change (Greenberg, 2007, pp. 415–416).

He recognizes the crucial functions of the clinician's presence, acceptance, attunement, and empathy; the establishment of a collaborative alliance; exploration of emotional experience, the origins and dynamics of feelings, and defensive processes; encouragement to accept emotions for the knowledge and understanding they provide; and the symbolization of emotion that underlies the creation of new meaning, narratives, and life stories (Greenberg, 2016).

The clinician and the patient attend to moment-by-moment experiencing as they explore concerns, focusing on the "felt sense" of sensations and feelings, searching for emotional, cognitive, or behavioral "markers" that serve as the focus of intervention. The clinician guides the therapeutic process at points, selecting different methods in light of particular patterns of feeling, thought, or behavior (for a description of therapeutic tasks and techniques see Greenberg, 2016).

Greenberg outlines six principles of emotion processing, centering on 1) awareness of emotion and formulating what we sense or feel; 2) expression of emotion; 3) regulation of emotion; 4) reflection on experience; 5) transformation of emotion through emotion; and 6) "corrective experience of emotion" through in-vivo experiences in therapy and the outer world. The patient and therapist collaborate in efforts to symbolize the "bodily felt referents" of inner life, creating new meaning that shapes narrative accounts and life stories. The therapeutic process deepens awareness of emotion, creating meanings that strengthen the sense of self, guiding thinking and behavior (Greenberg, 2016).

Therapeutic Action

Although humanistic thinkers have drawn on a range of intellectual traditions in developing therapeutic approaches, they share orienting perspectives, basic assumptions, and essential concerns that shape understanding and practice.

Conceptions of motivation, development, and personality emphasize inherent capacities for growth and self-actualization. By virtue of being human, presumably, we are predisposed to generate enriching experience as we develop our potentialities, actualize the self, and fulfill our desire to live. Thinkers embrace a teleological perspective, emphasizing the formative influence of our anticipated sense of the future rather than the events of the past in shaping the course of development.

In accord with the above perspectives, practitioners reject objectivist conceptions of truth and embrace phenomenological approaches, proposing that the only sense of reality we can know comes through the authority of our experience. We create meaning and construct models of the world. As we see in constructivist versions of cognitive and psychodynamic therapy, clinicians assume that what we regard as "truth" is unique to the individual, carried in the coherence and meaning of particular accounts of experience and courses of action.

As in the psychodynamic paradigm, practitioners view the therapeutic relationship and intersubjective communication as crucial sources of experiencing, learning, and growth. Patients and therapists co-create conditions that foster the process of exploration and discovery, strengthening capacities for awareness and engaging the authority of self as they process their experience of inner life encompassing the domains of sensation, emotion, thought, and imagery. Rogers came to think of the relationship as the fundamental dynamic of change and growth, proposing that the conditions of empathy, unconditional regard, and authenticity are sufficient to release the self-actualizing tendency.

Although experiential practitioners recognize the healing functions of the therapeutic relationship, they depart from the non-directive stance of Rogers and employ a range of methods drawn from psychodynamic, cognitive, and behavioral schools of thought. Client-centered and experiential therapists increasingly recognize the role of emotion in change and growth following developments in affective neuroscience and interpersonal neurobiology.

Clinicians assume that the dynamics of interaction foster the construction of new meaning and understanding as patients explore the bodily felt referents to problems in living and symbolize subjective experience through language. In accord with Dewey's pragmatic thought, concepts of therapeutic action recognize the functions of learning through experience that strengthens the sense of self and coping capacities (see Bohart & Watson, 2020, and Greenberg & Rice, 1997, for expanded accounts of experiential approaches).

There is a long tradition of empirical study in the humanistic paradigm, dating back to Rogers' pioneering studies in the 1950s. Clinical researchers have continued to document the efficacy and effectiveness of person-centered and experiential approaches. Although a review of the empirical literature is beyond the scope of this chapter, clinical scholars provide careful accounts of process and outcome research (for review of empirical studies and meta-analyses see Bohart & Watson, 2020; Elliott, Bohart, Watson & Murphy, 2018).

Neuroscience and Therapeutic Action

As in the psychodynamic tradition and constructivist versions of the cognitive paradigm, thinkers emphasize the crucial functions of the therapeutic relationship, open-ended dialogue, and interactive experience. In the field of interpersonal neurobiology, as discussed, clinical scholars have proposed that the presence of the practitioner and the patient's experience of synchrony, acceptance, support, and understanding in the therapeutic relationship facilitate the expression of emotion, helping one relinquish defensive patterns of behavior and rigid perceptions of self and others, exploring aspects of experience that have been distorted, denied, or dissociated (Cozolino, 2017).

In accord with Schore's formulations of right brain functions and therapeutic action, Rogers, Gendlin, and Greenberg emphasize the crucial importance of intersubjective communication and synchrony in regulating emotion and states of self, emphasizing the non-verbal elements of language—intonation, inflection, tone, pitch, force, and rhythm—as well as body movement, posture, gesture, and facial expression.

In Greenberg's conceptions of "therapeutic presence" the clinician is "fully in the moment on a multitude of levels, physically, emotionally, cognitively, spiritually, and relationally. The experience of therapeutic presence," he explains, involves "(a) being in contact with one's integrated and healthy self," while "(b) being open and receptive, to what is poignant in the moment and immersed in it," and "(c) with a larger sense of spaciousness and expansion of awareness and perception. This grounded, immersed, and expanded awareness occurs with the intention of being with and for the client, in service of his or her healing processes" (Greenberg, 2014, p. 353). At the most fundamental level, as Schore observes, the intersubjective process of therapy is determined not by what the clinician says or does; the key mechanism of change and growth, mediated by the functions of the right hemisphere, is "*how to be with the patient*" (Schore, 2019, p. 198).

Presumably, the patient comes to experience a wider range of emotion over the course of the therapeutic process, making feelings more available for reorganization, fostering integration of neural networks. The non-directive methods of the person-centered approach potentially help individuals engage executive functions and reflective capacities. The clinician's empathic reflection and validation of the patient's communications and exploration of concerns strengthens capacities to formulate and integrate experience.

As discussed in Chapter 3, conditions of mild to moderate arousal are thought to activate the production of neurotransmitters and neural growth hormones that govern the mechanisms of long-term potentiation, learning, and cortical reorganization. Clinicians who adopt a more active, directive approach, following the experiential approaches of Gendlin and Greenberg, potentially intensify emotion as they explore the dynamics of inner life and interactive experience, bringing challenge that carries implications for change. In focusing on features of inner life or outer experience that patients have failed to recognize or avoided out of fear or restrictions of opportunity, clinicians encourage the individual to experience, process, and express a wider range of feelings

From the perspective of neuroscience, we assume that experiential approaches carry the potential to foster integration of neural structures and functions across the domains of sensation, emotion, imagery, cognition, and behavior. The therapeutic process engages the verbal, analytic processes of the left hemisphere as the patient and therapist render experience into words and elaborate accounts of concerns, activating the mechanisms of "top-down" integration. As David Wallin explains: "Asking our patients to label what they feel in their bodies enlists cortical capacities in the processing of painful subcortical (i.e., somatic/affective) experience" (2007, p. 81).

Somatic approaches, engaging the breath, movement, or meditation, activate "bottom-up" forms of integration focused on the interoceptive experience of the body, engaging subcortical structures and the mechanisms of the right hemisphere, strengthening capacities for emotional regulation and coping. Growing awareness of bodily experience and processing of inner life strengthen the ability to tolerate painful states that have been managed through dissociation or other defensive processes.

The dynamics of narration engage the core structures of the brain, as noted above, synthesizing our experience of sensation, emotion, imagery, thought, and memory as we elaborate accounts of experience, fostering integration of neural networks throughout the cortical and subcortical regions. Although the person-centered approach does not emphasize concepts of narrative in classical formulations of therapeutic action, Rogers recognized the crucial role of language and meaning in change and growth. Clinical scholars in the experiential tradition have increasingly focused on narrative process and the ways in which the patient and therapist co-create accounts of self, life experience, and anticipated future (see for example Greenberg, 2016).

Concluding Comments

As we have seen, a range of intellectual traditions have shaped understanding and practice in the humanistic paradigm, encompassing phenomenological, existential, psychoanalytic, constructivist, and experiential perspectives. More recent formulations of therapeutic action have drawn on the fields of affective neuroscience and interpersonal neurobiology, emphasizing the dynamics of the therapeutic relationship, emotion, meaning, and experiential learning thought to bring about change and growth.

Clinical scholars continue to engage essential concerns that converge with the pragmatic thought of James and Dewey and the principles and values of clinical pragmatism, emphasizing the individuality and subjectivity of the person; notions of agency, intention, and will; exercise of freedom and choice; the crucial role of the therapeutic relationship, collaboration, and dialogue; co-creation of narrative and meaning; experiential learning; and inherent capacities for change, growth, and realization of potential in the individuation of the self. The focus is on the whole person, as human subject first and last—"the experiencing, active, living 'I'" (Sacks, 1984, p. 177).

References

Barzun, J. (2000). *From dawn to decadence.* New York: Harper Collins.

Binswanger, L. (1951/1963). *Being in the world* (J. Needleman, Trans.). New York: Basic Books.

Bohart, A. & Watson, J. (2011). Person centered and related experiential approaches, in S. Messer & A. Gurman (Eds.), *Essential psychotherapies* (pp. 223–260). New York: Guilford.

Bohart, A. & Watson, J. (2020). Person-centered and emotion-focused psychotherapies, in Messer, S. & Kaslow, N. (Eds.), *Essential psychotherapies* (pp. 221–256). New York: Guilford.

Boss, M. (1957/1963). *Psychoanalysis and daseinanalysis* (L. B. Lefebre, Trans.). New York. Basic Books.

Cozolino, L. (2017). *The neuroscience of psychotherapy*, 3rd edn. New York: Norton.

Elliot, R., Bohart, A., Watson, J. & Murphy, D. (2018). Therapist empathy and client outcome: An updated meta-analysis. *Psychotherapy*, 55 (4), 399–410.

Frankl, V. (1963). *Man's search for meaning: An introduction to logotherapy.* New York: Pocket Books.

Gendlin, E. (1962). *Experiencing and the creation of meaning.* Glencoe, IL: Free Press.

Gendlin, E. (1964). A theory of personality change, in P. Worchel & D. Byrne (Eds.), *Personality Change* (pp. 102–148). New York: Wiley.

Gendlin, E. (1991). On emotion in therapy, in J. Safran & L. Greenberg (Eds.), *Emotion, psychotherapy, and change* (pp. 255–279). New York: Guilford.

Gendlin, E. (1996). *Focusing-oriented psychotherapy.* New York: Guilford.

Goldstein, K. (1934/1995). *The organism.* New York: Zone Books.

Greenberg, L. (2007). Emotion coming of age. *Clinical Psychology Science and Practice*, 14, 414–421.

Greenberg, L. (2014). The therapeutic relationship in emotion-focused therapy. *Psychotherapy*, 51, 350–357.

Greenberg, L. (2016). *Emotion-focused therapy.* Washington, DC: American Psychological Association.

Greenberg, L. & Rice, L. (1997). Humanistic approaches to psychotherapy, in P. Wachel & S. Messer (Eds.), *Theories of psychotherapy: Origins and evolution* (pp. 97–129). Washington, DC: American Psychological Association.

Heidegger, M. (1962). *Being and time* (J. Macquarrie & E. Robinson, Trans.). New York: Basic Books.

Horney, K. (1942). *Self analysis.* New York: Norton.

Horney, K. (1950). *Neurosis and human growth.* New York: Norton.

Husserl, E. (1913/1962). *Ideas: General introduction to pure phenomenology* (W. R. Boyce, Trans.). New York: Collier.

166   *Clinical Theories and Therapeutic Action*

James, W. (1890). *Principles of psychology* (2 Vols.). New York: Holt.
James, W. (1911/1979). *Some problems of philosophy.* Cambridge, MA: Harvard University Press.
Kierkegaard, S. (1844/1944). *The concept of dread* (W. Lowrie, Trans.). Princeton, NJ: Princeton University Press.
Kirschenbaum, (2009). *Life and work of Carl Rogers.* Alexandria, VA: American Counseling Association.
Maslow, A. (1967a). A theory of metamotivation: The biological rooting of the value of life. *Journal of Humanistic Psychology,* 7, 93–127. Maslow, A. (1967b). Neurosis as a failure of personal growth. *Humanitas,* 3, 153–170.
Maslow, A. (1968). *Toward a psychology of being,* 2nd edn. Princeton, NJ: Van Nostrand.
Maslow, A. (1970). *Motivation and personality,* 2nd edn. New York: Harper.
Maslow, A. (1971). *The farther researches of human nature.* New York: Viking.
May, R. (1950/1977). *The meaning of anxiety.* New York: Norton.
Messer, S. & Kaslow, N. (Eds.). (2020). *Essential psychotherapies.* New York: Guilford.
Nietzsche, F. (1889/1982). Twilight of the idols, in W. Kaufmann (Ed.), *The portable Nietzsche.* New York: Penguin.
Perls, F. (1947). *Ego, hunger, and aggression.* London: Allen & Unwin.
Perls, F., Hefferline, R. & Goodman, P. (1951). *Gestalt therapy.* New York: Julian Press.
Rice, L. N. (1992). From naturalistic observation of psychotherapy process to micro theories of change, in Toukmanian, S. & Rennie, D. (Eds.), *Psychotherapy process research: Paradigmatic and narrative approaches* (pp. 1–21). Newbury Park, CA: Sage.
Rice, L. N. & Greenberg, L. (Eds.) (1984). *Patterns of change: Intensive analysis of psychotherapy process.* New York: Guilford.
Rogers, C. T. (1942). *Counseling and psychotherapy.* Boston, MA: Houghton-Mifflin.
Rogers, C. T. (1951/1965). *Client-centered therapy: Its current practice, implications, and theory.* Boston, MA: Houghton-Mifflin.
Rogers, C. T. (1957). The necessary and sufficient conditions of therapeutic personality change. *Journal of Consulting Psychology,* 21, 95–103.
Rogers, C. T. (1958a). A process conception of psychotherapy. *American Psychologist,* 13, 142–149.
Rogers, C. T. (1958b). The characteristics of a helping relationship, in C. T. Rogers, *On becoming a person* (pp. 39–58). Boston, MA: Houghton-Mifflin.
Rogers, C. T. (1959). A theory of therapy, personality, and interpersonal relationships, as developed in the client-centered framework, in Koch, S. (Ed.), *Psychology: A study of a science,* Vol. 3 (pp. 184–256). New York: McGraw Hill.
Rogers, C. T. (1961). *On becoming a person.* Boston, MA: Houghton-Mifflin.
Sacks, O. (1984). *A leg to stand on.* New York: Simon & Schuster.
Schore, A. (2019). *Right brain psychotherapy.* New York: Norton.
Siegel, D. (2018). *Mind.* New York: Norton.
Siegel, D. (2020). *The developing mind,* 3rd edn. New York: Guilford.
Wallin, D. (2007). *Attachment in psychotherapy.* New York: Guilford.
Yalom, I. (1980). *Existential psychotherapy.* New York: Basic Books.

9 Clinical Pragmatism and Therapeutic Action

The ultimate compliment is to be found and used...

–D. W. Winnicott

Researchers speak of "the dynamics of neuroplasticity" and the "mechanisms of therapeutic action" in their writings on change and growth, but we rediscover the voice of our patients in the clinical situation, joining language and life, speaking of "experiencing," "feeling," "willing," and "acting" as they negotiate problems in living. In embracing the values of clinical pragmatism, as we have seen, we focus on our patients as subjects, exploring the phenomenal realms of lived experience, working to understand the nature of their suffering, worries, hopes, and prospects—what, now, is the matter and what carries the potential to help. We think of psychotherapy as an open practice, emphasizing the crucial role of the relationship, collaboration, dialogue, narrative, and experiential learning, and we assume that beneficial outcomes follow from flexible use of different formulations, approaches and methods as we carry out "experiments in adapting to need."

In this chapter I present two cases and show how the principles of pragmatic thought deepen our appreciation of essential concerns in the clinical situation, emphasizing the importance of idiographic approaches and the practical outcomes of ideas and methods over the course of the therapeutic process. The pluralist orientation of clinical pragmatism, encompassing scientific and humanistic domains of understanding, makes the multiplicity of approaches a defining feature of therapeutic practice. The cases illustrate the challenges we face as we negotiate tensions between particular approaches and alternative points of view in our conceptions of therapeutic action, change, and growth.

Case 1: Jonathan

Jonathan, age 28, developed diffuse anxiety, panic attacks, and dissociative states 18 months after he was critically injured in an explosion during military service in Iraq. He had suffered a severe concussion, internal injuries, and multiple fractures of the spinal cord and both legs, and was left with hearing loss and chronic pain after back and leg surgeries. In addition to the injuries that he had suffered in the explosion, he had witnessed the deaths of civilians and soldiers over the course of his service. He had completed an intensive course of rehabilitation in a military medical center after his recovery from life-threatening injuries and developed the above symptoms after returning to his childhood home, where he lived with his aunt. He was frightened by the sudden onset and intensity of his symptoms, unable to make sense of his experience.

Beyond the physical injuries and traumatic events that he related in the accounts of his experience in Iraq, other sources of vulnerability emerged in his developmental history. His mother, divorced shortly after his birth, had died suddenly when he was 6, following a dissecting aortal aneurism, and he and his older brother were placed in foster care. Nearly two years later they were adopted by their aunt, his mother's younger sister. They lived in one of the most blighted neighborhoods of Chicago, an African-American community increasingly fragmented by warring gangs, violence, and crime, but his aunt took them to the botanic garden near their home every Sunday after church where they spent the afternoon playing in the park.

Jonathan developed a deep love for his aunt, who taught kindergarten in the public school system. She appears to have been taxed beyond the bounds of what she could manage, however, and he recalled fears that she, too, would suddenly die. She helped him with his homework, as he struggled in school, and he developed an interest in math and computers, hoping to begin an apprenticeship program in information technology following graduation from high school. He changed his plans at the start of his senior year, he explained, after his brother was killed by a stray bullet in a gang shooting. He joined the army, in search of a new life. He served in the infantry, attending an advanced training school before he was deployed to Iraq, and had found a sense of belonging, meaning, and purpose in the military.

The vulnerability and dependency that he had experienced over the course of care in the rehabilitation program appeared to have intensified needs for closeness and connection after his return, but he found himself avoiding contact with family members, fearful that they would press him to talk about the course of events in Iraq. He had come to feel a growing sense of hopelessness, helplessness, and dread—"like something bad is always about to happen"—and described a range of problems in functioning that met diagnostic criteria for post-traumatic stress disorder. He also showed signs of post-concussion syndrome, including lapses in attention, concentration, and memory, difficulties putting thoughts into words, sensitivity to light and noise, and fatigue.

He had begun a course of antidepressant medication, following consultations with a psychiatrist and neurologist in a military medical center, and reported some improvement in symptoms. He was exploring options for services through the Vocational Rehabilitation and Employment program of the federal government, hopeful that he would be able to arrange on-the-job training in the field of information technology and find an accommodating work environment. The psychiatrist encouraged him to consider a course of psychotherapy, believing it would help him process his experience of trauma and negotiate the challenges of his transition from military service to independent living.

I began to meet with Jonathan weekly in the community clinic where I carried out my practice. I realized that his current range of functioning, compromised by the traumatic brain injury and extended periods of panic, fragmentation, and dissociation, and the history of early loss, disruptions in caretaking, patterns of attachment, and trauma potentially limited his ability to form an alliance and make use of the therapeutic process. I followed his lead as he related the course of his experience, working to understand why, now, he found himself overcome by dread, unable to eat or sleep, fearful to leave the surrounds of his home. As he described his symptoms I related them to our understanding of post-traumatic stress disorder and post-concussion syndrome, reviewing the dynamics of hyperarousal, numbing, and avoidance, working to create a heuristic that would help him make sense of his experience.

The nature of his symptoms would have led many clinicians to initiate a standard course of cognitive-behavioral therapy at the outset, following evidence-based guidelines for treatment of post-traumatic stress disorder, but such a nomothetic approach in itself would have been reductive in light of the wider range of concerns that Jonathan related over the course of the consultation and the global compromise in functioning that likely would have limited his ability to make use of technical procedures or skills training. I feared that any standardized course of treatment would have intensified his experience of limitation and loss. Above all, I thought it was crucial to establish the therapeutic relationship and begin to co-create a holding environment that would allow us to explore options for treatment of specific symptoms and emerging concerns in light of his current capacities and range of functioning.

As we have seen, psychodynamic perspectives emphasize the sustaining functions of the therapeutic relationship and the constancy of care in the holding environment. We realize the crucial role of empathic attunement, synchrony, and repair following breaks in the continuity of interactive experience, focusing on the non-verbal, right-brain dominated aspects of the therapeutic relationship that we register through what we sense, feel, and do rather than through what we say.

I attended closely to Jonathan's experience of our interaction and the surrounds of the clinic as he related the course of his symptoms and concerns, working to provide the constancy of care that Winnicott describes in his conceptions of holding. He was particularly reactive to bright light, sudden noise, and the scents of cleaning products that we would relate to implicit memories of his experience in Iraq. I attempted to reduce stimuli that carried the potential to intensify fear or activate dissociative states in the therapeutic setting. We pulled the blinds to filter the morning sun and used white noise to limit the impingements of unexpected sound. He experienced chronic pain in his legs and back, and we rearranged cushions to help him feel as comfortable as possible. He sometimes stood to ease the pain, walking back and forth.

His experience of my presence, acceptance, attunement, and concern appeared to foster the development of the therapeutic alliance and the holding environment, facilitating our efforts to explore the dynamics of problems in functioning, formulate goals, and think about the course of help and care. In accord with findings in the field of interpersonal neurobiology, I realized that our ways of being together and interactive forms of communication, mediated largely by the functions of the right hemisphere, carried the potential to help him strengthen capacities to regulate emotion and restore cohesion in sense of self following periods of fragmentation and dissociative states. (Recall Allan Schore's formulations of right-brain interactive experience and therapeutic action reviewed in Chapters 2, 3, and 5, and Carl Rogers' formulations of "psychological contact" and Leslie Greenberg's accounts of "therapeutic presence," described in Chapter 8).

Although Jonathan struggled with a range of problems in functioning, he found himself disabled by his experience of panic—"frozen," he explained, unable to carry out the activities of everyday life. The beginning phase of our work, accordingly, focused on ways of managing his experience of fear. His sudden episodes of panic were associated with a range of symptoms, including sensations of choking, shortness of breath, chest pain, palpitations, sweating, numbness, nausea, vertigo, and feelings of unreality; at points he feared he would die. I drew on standardized protocols for treatment of panic disorder as we proceeded, selectively integrating educational, cognitive, and behavioral approaches developed over the course of clinical research (see Barlow, Allen & Basden, 2007). We reviewed the dynamics of his physiological reactions, thinking of the panic attacks as a "misfiring" of the sympathetic nervous system, precipitating the full-blown fight or flight response. I shared my understanding of the ways in which fear compromises executive functions, limiting our capacities to process experience and cope.

I drew on a range of concepts and methods developed in the third wave models of cognitive-behavioral therapy in an effort to help him begin to shift the way he related to his experience of fear, focusing on the development of capacities to actively engage, observe, and accept the flow of the sensations, feelings, and thoughts rather than trying to avoid, challenge, or escape them. In accord with fundamental concepts of therapeutic action, our goal was to change the context in which he experienced fear and panic, coming to recognize sensations, feelings, and thoughts as transitory phenomena rather than as fixed realities that represented the totality of his experience. I outlined basic breathing exercises that carried the potential to help him manage his symptoms, engaging "bottom-up" mechanisms of re-regulation.

As discussed in Chapter 3, the middle prefrontal region of the brain is instrumental in emotional regulation, integrating information across core structures, while the dorsolateral area, associated with the "rational mind," is specialized for conscious, verbal processing of experience. Accordingly, as David Wallin explains, "simply thinking aloud about difficult emotions with our patients—particularly traumatized patients—may be useful... but insufficient"

(2007, p. 81). What is crucial is activating the middle prefrontal cortex by helping patients process their experience of sensation and emotion in real time. The focus on bodily experience and on breathing can strengthen capacities for emotional regulation and management of the dynamics of inner life.

As Wallin observes: "This interoceptive attention is a form of mindfulness that helps ground patients in the present moment, potentially modulating the distress associated with the traumatic past and feared future" (2007, p. 81). As patients find the words to formulate their experience of sensation and emotion they activate cortical capacities in processing subcortical realms of experience. Deepened awareness of somatic experience and incremental efforts to tolerate overwhelming emotion prepares patients to more fully process and integrate previously dissociated feelings, thoughts, images, and memories.

Although Jonathan's continued experience of anxiety, fragmentation, and dissociation limited his capacities to make use of cognitive and behavioral methods in the first phase of therapy, he came to view his recurring experiences of fear and panic as occasions to strengthen the development of coping skills—a shift in perspective he introduced that appeared to deepen his sense of agency, challenge, and mastery.

His experience of dread and panic fluctuated with sudden drops into pockets of dissociation and numbing in the middle phase of therapy as we began to explore the course of traumatic events in Iraq. He had found himself unable to relate memories of what he had witnessed at the start of our work, fearful that he could not manage his emotions, but he increasingly felt the need "to find the words" to describe events he had not shared with others, including the injuries and deaths of fellow soldiers as convoys were hit by improvised explosive devices. I spoke of the ways in which the sensations, emotions, and thoughts associated with trauma are split off from awareness, encapsulated as frozen fragments—"splinter psyches," as Jung called them, carried as implicit memory.

As discussed in Chapters 2 and 3, researchers propose that ongoing engagement of sensation, emotion, and cognition over the course of the therapeutic process fosters the reorganization of under-integrated and under-regulated neural networks believed to perpetuate dissociation and dysfunction. As we return to various aspects of traumatic experience, presumably, we activate neural firing associated with earlier events, creating new synaptic connections, reorganizing neural networks. If we think of dissociation as the fundamental problem of trauma, as Jung proposed, the aim of therapy is association—integrating the split-off elements of traumatic experience into our ongoing sense of self and life story so that we come to realize "that was then, and this is now" (Van der Kolk, 2014, p. 183).

Object relations formulations guided our exploration of the ways in which working models of self and relational life had influenced his perceptions of traumatic experience, current relationships, and patterns of interaction in the therapeutic relationship, including transference reactions. As a child Jonathan had come to experience his needs as a burden, following the death of his mother, his placement in foster care, and the adoption by his aunt, fearful that she, like his mother, would die suddenly. Our exploration of interactive experience in the therapeutic situation revealed that he feared the accounts of his experience in Iraq would also overwhelm me. Enactments and the dynamics of transference and counter-transference reactions served as crucial sources of experiencing and understanding as we processed less conscious elements of his trauma and strengthened his capacities to formulate and share his experience of vulnerability and need with me and family members, realizing that he did not have to protect others from himself.

We drew on the methods of classical cognitive therapy in efforts to challenge vicious circles of thought, feeling, and action ("My life is over," "I'm broken," "Nobody really wants to spend time with me") and take more full account of actual circumstances and realistic prospects. He had come to experience the world as a dangerous place, restricting patterns of activity, avoiding opportunities to engage extended family in spite of his longings for closeness and connection. Following the basic principles of behavioral activation, we identified tasks that provided occasions for him to challenge his avoidance of experience, enlarge ranges of activity, and engage relational life in light of essential concerns and goals, creating sources of positive reinforcement. I accompanied him on a return to the botanical gardens where he had spent Sunday afternoons with his aunt and brother, and he began taking weekly walks in the park, finding comfort and restoration in the experience of nature (see Sacks, 2019, for an account of "hortophilia" and the therapeutic functions of nature).

As he continued to relate accounts of events in the middle phase of therapy, recounting the particular details of his experience, expanding earlier reports of what had happened, his fear receded and he found himself increasingly able to manage his symptoms of anxiety and dissociative states, making more full use of cognitive techniques and breathing practices. From the perspective of the behavioral paradigm we can think of our repeated exploration of sensations, feelings, thoughts, and images associated with events as a form of in-vivo exposure. He was able to experience and integrate aspects of inner life that he had avoided out of fear. (Recall Wachtel's formulations of exposure outlined in Chapter 6). From a psychoanalytic perspective, we can characterize this phase of our work as the process of "remembering, repeating, and working through" that Freud describes in his classic formulations of therapeutic action and change, facilitating the reorganization and integration of neural networks (see Chapter 4).

Traumatic experience threatens basic assumptions about the resilience and worthiness of the self and challenges fundamental conceptions of meaning and justice. In the face of adversity, the assumptive world that has given us a sense of coherence and continuity may be taxed beyond the range of its adaptive function, leading to disorganization and the onset of post-traumatic stress disorder. Inevitably, the effort to restore a sense of order and meaning assumes the form of narrative: stories are ways of organizing experience, interpreting events, and restoring the sense of self, identity, and the assumptive world.

Jonathan began to review the course of his life as we entered the fourth year of therapy, coming to understand earlier events in a new light. The dynamics of narration are thought to engage the core structures of the brain, as discussed in Chapter 3, synthesizing our experience of sensation, emotion, imagery, thought, and memory as we elaborate accounts of events, fostering integration of neural networks throughout the cortical and subcortical regions. I had studied classics in college, and I found myself beginning to make connections between the stories he related and accounts of war and loss in ancient Greek theater. The tragedies may have functioned as a ritual reintegration for combat veterans, as Bessel Van der Kolk notes, providing occasions for catharsis and healing. Peter Sellers was directing a production of Handel's *Hercules* at the Lyric Opera in Chicago at the time, and he organized a discussion of the work with a group of veterans from the community. Jonathan attended the program, deeply moved as fellow veterans shared their stories, bearing witness to the experience of war, trauma, and loss.

Psychodynamic understanding continued to guide our exploration of the ways in which earlier patterns of care, relational life, social surrounds, trauma, and loss had shaped the course of his life, influencing ways of being, relating, and coping. We explored the meaning of traumatic events in Iraq in light of his earlier experience of loss, connecting the sudden onset of symptoms after the return to his childhood home to the tragic deaths of his mother and brother. He was increasingly able to make sense of his symptoms in view of the losses, exploring the meaning and implications of events, working to clarify essential concerns as he elaborated his personal narrative and life story. Humanistic perspectives guided our exploration of existential concerns.

Jonathan decided to end the course of his therapy, carried out over seven years, after he accepted a position with the human service organization that had sponsored his on-the-job training program. He had deepened his sense of connection and closeness with extended family and was beginning to form friendships. He continued to live with his aunt, exploring shared interests in urban gardening, moving into what he came to call his "second life." Over the years he has returned for brief courses of therapy at symptomatic junctures, continuing to negotiate emerging concerns, challenges, and possibilities.

Case 2: Marta

> "You are my toy," Marta announced at the start of our consultation. "You move when I want you to move, and you speak when I want you to speak... If you don't do what I want," she challenged, "what good are you?"
>
> "Useless," I found myself saying. "We will have to find out if I can be useful."

Marta, approaching her 30th birthday, had been referred to me by a social worker in a community mental health center where she had received psychiatric care for more than a decade. She was thought to be autistic as a child and diagnosed as schizophrenic in adolescence; more recently, social workers had documented a range of problems in functioning encompassed in reformulations of borderline personality disorder, emphasizing her inability to regulate emotion, control behavior, and negotiate relational life.

I learned that she had been born in a state psychiatric hospital and placed in foster care after her mother, believed to be schizophrenic, was unable to care for her. She had had a succession of foster care arrangements through childhood and had been placed in residential treatment as an adolescent. She was hospitalized at the age of 16, after a suicide attempt, and had been followed by a series of psychiatrists in the mental health center for pharmacotherapy and supportive care. She had found antipsychotic and antidepressant medication helpful, over the years, and was completing a psychiatric rehabilitation program affiliated with a university medical center, preparing to begin work as a data entry clerk. She had been unsuccessful in her earlier attempts to carry out psychotherapy in light of her disruptive behavior, and unable to form an alliance with a series of clinicians, but her case manager explained that she was reconsidering the possibility of therapy as she anticipated the transition to full-time employment and independent living.

I would follow Marta in intensive psychotherapy for more than a decade. In this account I show how the developmental psychology of Donald Winnicott served as an orienting perspective for therapeutic action that allowed us to integrate a range of approaches and methods over the course of our work. His conceptions of trauma, developmental arrest, and the maturational process shaped my understanding of essential concerns as we carried out pragmatic "experiments in adapting to need."

Winnicott believes that we are born with an inherent drive to actualize the "true self," the inviolate core of our being, and he describes the "maturational process" that governs the course of development. When caretakers fail to provide a good enough holding environment at the start of life, however, our sense of "going on being" is disrupted and we are thrown into chaos. In light of my understanding of Marta's history and the etiology of borderline personality disorder, I assumed that genetic factors and traumatic conditions over the course of care in infancy and early childhood had compromised the dynamics of neural integration and the establishment of a core sense of self, leading to developmental arrest, predisposing her to a range of problems in functioning. Neuropsychological testing had shown deficits in executive function, attention, and memory consistent with a large body of research documenting altered patterns of brain maturation in borderline disorders (see Cozolino, 2017, for reviews of empirical findings).

Like many patients diagnosed with borderline personality disorder, she struggled to preserve cohesion in sense of self and identity, unable to regulate her experience of sensation, feeling, and behavior. Her capacity to tolerate distress was limited and she was slow to restore equilibrium following periods of disorganization and dysregulation. Over the years she had cut herself frequently, threatened suicide, and used alcohol and marijuana to regulate her feelings. She had developed ways of managing self-destructive behaviors over the course of her rehabilitation program, drawing on the methods of dialectical behavior therapy, but she found herself overwhelmed by emotion much of the time, caught in vicious circles of feeling, thought, and action. She continued to experience transient psychotic symptoms and extended periods of dissociation, relying on what Winnicott describes as "omnipotent defenses" in efforts to manage "unimaginable terrors"—fears of "going to pieces" (Winnicott, 1960/ 1965, p. 47).

Although radical lapses and failings in care may undermine the integrative functions of the maturational process, Winnicott believes that we continue to search for conditions that carry the potential to reinstate the course of development, engaging the dynamics of "going on being" instrumental in the emergence of the self as subject—what he calls the experience of "I-ness:" "I am, I exist, I gather experiences and enrich myself... and have interaction with the not-me, the actual world of shared reality" (1962/1965, p. 61).

In accord with his faith in our capacities for development, Winnicott assumes that the patient structures the therapeutic situation to recreate conditions that were compromised in earlier caretaking and reinstate the process of "going on being," fostering the integration of the self. He compares the fundamental provisions of holding in infancy to ways of being in the therapeutic situation, emphasizing the crucial functions of the clinician's presence, acceptance, attunement, and responsiveness, joining the patient as they co-create moments of meeting that open new possibilities; the "ultimate compliment," Winnicott writes, "is to be found and used" (1968/1987, p. 103; see Borden, 2009, for expanded accounts of Winnicott's developmental psychology).

I began seeing Marta twice a week in the community clinic where I carried out my practice. I followed her lead as we began our work, finding myself challenged, like earlier therapists, in our efforts to form an alliance and establish the holding environment. She sat in silence, watching me, seemingly transfixed, unable to find the words to say what had moved her to begin yet another attempt at therapy, irritated by my expressions of concern, interest, and support.

Language is a core constituent of neural and psychological development, instrumental in the formation of memory and identity, but Marta was unable to provide a coherent account of her life. She had little memory of her childhood or adolescence, she told me, and no interest in exploring the course of her earlier experience: "It was what it was." She experienced fluctuating states of dread, anger, deadness, emptiness, helplessness, and hopelessness as we began our work, finding me "useless," "a deadbeat," like her earlier therapists. At other times, however, I found that she was able to focus on the concerns of everyday life and register her experience of my care and efforts to help as she shared her worries, engaged in the therapeutic process, seemingly feeling a sense of hope and possibility.

I functioned as a case manager much of the time, providing information, advice, and guidance as she moved from a single room occupancy housing arrangement to a studio apartment, settled into a new neighborhood, and began to carry out the activities of her new job. We talked about the concrete particulars of shopping, cooking, housekeeping, and domestic life. I helped her negotiate bus routes as she found her way around the city from her new home. Winnicott's accounts of case management, emphasizing the ways in which concrete forms of help potentially foster change and growth, deepened my appreciation of the critical functions of instrumental activities, often seen as extrinsic to the therapeutic process (see Kantor, 1990; Winnicott, 1963/ 1965). There were good days and bad days, good moments and bad moments, as we continued our work.

The mental operations of splitting generated distinct qualities of experience in the first phase of the therapy, and there was no middle ground between good and bad. Most of the time Marta felt a pervasive sense of agitation, anger, and destructiveness that she was unable to relate to the dynamics of inner life or outer circumstances; we could not identify the precipitating conditions. She saw herself and me as bad—"evil"—in these states and showed no capacity to summon alternative views of either of us as good. When she identified with the experience of herself as good, however, she found me caring, supportive, and helpful, and had no memory of having felt otherwise. She was unable to connect these radically different experiences of herself, others, and the world. We came to speak of the fluctuations as her "inner weather," shaping ongoing experiences of herself, others, and world.

Marta had not developed the capacity to process or formulate internal states of herself as a subject, reflect on her behavior, or consider different ways of seeing, understanding, and acting as she related the course of her days. It was as if she were devoid of subjectivity, not having established a core sense of self, unable to experience herself as an agent. She seldom used personal pronouns or active verbs in her speech. For example, rather than saying, "I'm having a hard day and I feel bad," she would say "it bad today… hate it… everything bad." There was no distinction, seemingly, between perception and interpretation of events in such non-reflective states; it was the realm of things as they were—good or bad—and it seemed crucial that only one emotional plane exist at a time. In the absence of a reflective self, she lived in a surround shaped by actions rather than thoughts, words, or reflection (see Ogden, 1986; Wallin, 2007, p. 239).

From the perspective of Winnicott's developmental psychology, I came to understand that Marta experienced me as a "subjective object" over the first phase of our work, unable to engage me as a distinct, independent person beyond the bounds of her inner life, relating to me largely through the dynamics of projection and omnipotence, speaking and acting as if she were in possession and control of me and the world. "You're not human," she continued to tell me. "You're my toy… You speak when I want you to speak… you move when I want you to move… humans have feelings… I don't have feelings."

What matters most at this point in the therapeutic process, Winnicott emphasizes, is not what we say but what we do. The concrete help that I provided in my role as case manager continued to strengthen the therapeutic alliance and the constancy of care in the holding environment. Crucially, I did not challenge her renderings of me as an object, "a toy," an elaboration of inner world. I felt I must accept her as she was, without imposing any need to change herself. Following Winnicott's formulations of therapeutic action, I remained steadfast and joined her, co-creating ways of being together that carried the potential to reinstate the maturational process. Our task was to fashion a facilitating environment and co-create conditions that would allow her to go about the business of being herself, providing "environmental adaptations" that she had presumably lacked in the course of her development (see Winnicott, 1960/1965).

In doing so, however, it was critical that I preserve the deeper structure of the therapeutic frame that made our ways of working possible, attending to boundaries and the concrete details of care. I set limits as she repeatedly tested me in her expressions of anger and threats of suicide, telling her what I would and would not do in a given situation. I understood her behavior as enactments— forms of communication reflecting the depth of her despair and the hope that I could help her, allowing me to act decisively without threat of abandonment or punishment. As Winnicott emphasizes, "You accept hate and meet it with strength rather than revenge" (1963/1965, p. 229; see also 1947/1965). My willingness to struggle with Marta was essential. At this point in development, as David Wallin observes, the subjective realm is largely a world of physical action: if we can speak of a therapeutic dialogue, it is a dialogue of action (2007, pp. 239–240). Lacking the capacities for mentalization or reflection, Marta could tell the story of her experience only through enactments, not having fully established the capacity for symbolization and use of words.

As we moved into the fifth year of our work Marta was increasingly able to process her experience of splitting and contradictory states of mind, coming to realize the ways in which her fluctuating perceptions of others as good or bad perpetuated vicious circles of feeling, thought, and action. There were times, for example, when she experienced me as caring and helpful, grateful for my support and understanding, and there were times when she saw me as cold, uncaring, incompetent—"useless."

The repeated experience of strain, rupture, and repair over the course of our interaction provided crucial occasions for experiential learning as we explored the dynamics of underlying emotions, thoughts, and behavior. I drew on basic methods of dialectical behavior therapy as we continued to explore the realms of sensation and emotion, focusing on the development of skills that would strengthen her capacities to attend to experience, tolerate distress, and regulate emotion. More and more she came to embody, name, and share—rather than enact—what she was feeling, deepening her sense of agency, mastery, and self-esteem. In time, she would come to regard feelings as ways of knowing herself more deeply, more fully accepting herself as "human."

Marta discovered transitional phenomena and the experience of play in the holding environment of the therapeutic surround as we entered the eighth year of our work. One day she walked over to the book case and picked up a pot. "Look at this!" she exclaimed. "I made it! It's mine." She took the pot home, brought it back on her next visit, placed it on the book case, returned to it at the end of the session, and took it home again. She would repeat the ritual over the next year.

We had entered the realm of transitional phenomena that Winnicott describes in his developmental psychology (1971, 1988). In this "third region," bridging inner experience and outer realities, ongoing experiences of merger and separation establish the sense that what is needed can be created or found, fostering the emergence of capacities for "object use." The experience deepens the subject's sense of aliveness, as Michael Eigen observes, "opening the way for a new kind of freedom because one is coming to experience the other as real" (1981/1993, p. 112).

Marta continued to move out of the encapsulated world of omnipotent fantasy as we carried out our work, consolidating a core sense of self, increasingly able to relate to me as the "objective object" of Winnicott's developmental narrative. She came to experience me as real, distinct and separate from herself, as an individual with an independent center of feeling, thinking, initiative, and action, able to relate to me in our experience of similarity and difference. Her illusions of magical creation and control receded as she consolidated capacities to make use of my provisions—"reality presenting," in Winnicott's phrase—and engage in a back and forth with actual experience in the outer world. She was developing capacities for "I-ness" and object use— "other than me experience," as Winnicott thinks of it, deepening her sense of aliveness and strengthening her ability to engage in dialogue, negotiate the dynamics of relational life, and live in the world of others.

Discussion

The accounts of Jonathan and Marta, representative of many patients followed in community mental health clinics, deepen our appreciation of essential concerns in our conceptions of therapeutic action, help, and care. In this section I consider the course of our work in light of the orienting perspectives, values, and themes of clinical pragmatism introduced in Chapter 1.

Individuality, Subjectivity, and the Human Particularity of the Therapeutic Process

In following the basic principles and values of clinical pragmatism, as I have emphasized, we focus on the subjectivity of the individual and the unique circumstances of the clinical situation that defy classification, taking account of the complexities and contingencies that shape the course of the therapeutic process. We challenge a technical rationalism and reductive approaches to help and care based on rigid adherence to particular theories, empirical findings, methods, or procedures, rejecting views of practitioners as instrumental problem-solvers, realizing the limits of nomothetic models of treatment. As I show in the accounts of Jonathan and Marta, we co-create "experiments in adapting to need" in light of emerging concerns, goals, capacities, and skills, exploring the ways we make use of different elements over the course of the therapeutic process, embracing idiographic formulations of help and care as we discover what proves useful.

Relationship, Collaboration, and Interactive Experience

We recognize the crucial role of the therapeutic alliance, collaboration, and the functions of interactive experience in change and growth, realizing the critical importance of the bond between the clinician and the patient and their shared understanding of the goals and core activities of help and care. We carry out open-ended dialogue and emphasize the co-creation of narrative and meaning as we proceed, accepting the limits of our understanding, remaining open to the occasions of experiential learning that deepen insight and inform different ways of working.

As we have seen, the dynamics of interactive experience carry the potential to foster change in a variety of ways. In the domain of interpersonal neurobiology, we assume that the core conditions of the therapeutic relationship activate biological mechanisms that enhance neuroplasticity. The experience of synchrony and attunement and the constancy of care in the holding environment, mediated by right-brain modes of communication, strengthen internal functions instrumental in regulation of emotion and subjective states. New and different ways of relating are believed to reorganize networks of association across neural structures, including motives, emotions, and cognitions linked with representations of self and others, defensive processes, and behavior. Ongoing interaction facilitates efforts to process enactments and transference and countertransference states, deepen capacities for reflection, and develop more functional patterns of behavior through the dynamics of internalization, modeling, and experiential learning. The working alliance serves as a catalyst, helping the patient more fully engage the core activities of the therapeutic process and make use of enriching relationships, activities, and places in everyday life.

We revise understanding and action in light of evolving outcomes. Jonathan was able to reflect on his experience of the therapeutic process from the start of our work, sharing what he found helpful or limiting at particular points, and his ongoing accounts shaped the course of therapy as he explored concerns and expanded the range of his capacities and skills. Marta, in contrast, was limited in her ability to engage in dialogue or reflect on her experience of the therapeutic process as we began our work. If we could speak of a therapeutic dialogue, as I explain, it was a dialogue of action; she spoke through enactments of behavior. In time, as she consolidated a core sense of self, she developed the capacity to make use of words in the give and take of relational life, reflecting on her experience of the therapy, describing approaches and methods she found particularly helpful as she negotiated ongoing vulnerabilities and the challenges of everyday life.

Pluralist Orientation, Encompassing Scientific and Humanistic Domains of Understanding

In accord with the pluralist orientation of clinical pragmatism, we recognize the value of scientific and humanistic realms of understanding, considering a range of orienting perspectives, theories, empirical research, therapeutic languages, and models of intervention as we formulate our understanding of the case and consider potential courses of help and care.

In the domain of science, I drew on conceptual syntheses and empirical findings in the fields of interpersonal neurobiology, developmental psychopathology, and trauma as I carried out my work with Jonathan and Marta, taking account of biological factors as I formulated my understanding of vulnerability, problems in functioning, and therapeutic action. I reviewed research documenting the range of neurodevelopmental vulnerabilities associated with borderline personality disorder and post-traumatic stress disorder, realizing the potential benefits of pharmacological approaches, psychotherapy, and the experiential opportunities of everyday life believed to foster neural integration and strengthen capacities to regulate emotion, thought, and behavior.

I reviewed evidence-based protocols for treatment of post-traumatic stress disorder, panic disorder, and post-concussion syndrome in my work with Jonathan, selectively integrating concepts and methods from nomothetic models of intervention over the course of our work. I followed research on the etiology and treatment of borderline personality disorder over the course of my work with Marta, integrating methods from third-wave cognitive-behavioral models. Although scientific reasoning guided my ways of working in both cases, I avoided reductive or rigid applications of treatment guidelines or protocols, willing to forsake technical rigor in my efforts to help, trying to figure out what elements seemed sensible, valid, and useful.

In the realm of humanistic understanding, as discussed in earlier chapters, we focus on the individuality of the person and subjective experience; notions of personal agency, intention and will; exercise of freedom and choice; the co-creation of narrative and meaning, and inherent capacities for change, growth, and realization of potential. We think of the humanities as a foundation of practice, recognizing the ways in which the liberal arts enrich our faculties of reflection, imagination, emotion, and empathy. Stories help us appreciate the workings of fate, circumstance, and fortune that shape the course of our lives, as Jonathan found when he joined the group of veterans to discuss Handel's *Hercules* and the experience of war.

As we have seen, the foundational schools of psychotherapy differ in the philosophical perspectives, root metaphors, values, and methods that shape conceptions of therapeutic action, enlarging ways of attending, understanding, and acting. We must inevitably negotiate fundamental tensions between more pure conceptions of the therapeutic endeavor and more pragmatic renderings of help and care as we proceed with our practice.

From the perspective of clinical pragmatism, as I have shown in my accounts of both cases, we consider the perspectives of our purist thinkers selectively in light of changing needs, capacities, and circumstances, combining ideas and methods from divergent approaches that would be considered incompatible in more pure renderings of the therapeutic endeavor within the foundational schools of thought. I drew on ideas and methods from psychodynamic, behavioral, cognitive, and humanistic approaches over the course of my work with Jonathan and Marta, thinking of the therapeutic process as open-ended and provisional, guided by experiential learning and practical outcomes rather than by fixed commitments to particular theoretical perspectives, empirical findings, or technical strategies per se.

Therapeutic Action, Experiential Learning, and Practical Outcomes

We change over the course of psychotherapy, making use of different elements as we negotiate problems in living, deepen understanding, and strengthen capacities and skills. In working from a pragmatic perspective, as noted, we vary ways of working in light of emerging concerns, evolving circumstances, and the ongoing outcomes of experiential learning rather than applying a standardized model of intervention based on a diagnosis made at the start of treatment. In following the principles of clinical pragmatism, we emphasize process and context in our formulations of therapeutic action, change, and growth.

As I show in my accounts of Jonathan and Marta, different approaches proved more or less helpful at different points in the therapeutic process. At the start of our work Jonathan found himself compromised by a range of symptoms, limiting his ability to engage experiential opportunities that carried the potential to bring about change and growth. As we established the therapeutic alliance and the constancy of care in the holding environment, however, he was increasingly able to make use of cognitive and behavioral methods as he managed his experience of anxiety and panic; in time, he was able to engage a wider range of relationships, activities, and places that he had avoided out of fear. As he continued to restore a cohesive sense of self, he shifted the focus of our work from management of symptoms to his experience of trauma and loss, finding the words to form accounts of what had happened in Iraq, revising and expanding the narratives of his life story as he explored existential concerns. Psychodynamic, cognitive, and humanistic approaches served as orienting perspectives in the later phases of our work.

Winnicott's formulations of trauma, developmental arrest, and the maturational process offered a coherent way of understanding the course of Marta's experience as we began our consultations, providing a flexible, pragmatic framework for different ways of working over the course of the therapeutic process. I followed her lead, joining the instrumental activities of case management, the skills-based approaches of dialectical behavior therapy, and the relational perspectives that Winnicott had described in his case studies. Her capacity to make use of various approaches shaped the course of our work, in accord with his developmental perspective, guided by changing needs, experiential learning, and concrete outcomes.

Concluding Comments

If we are to avoid the dogmatic embrace of a purist paradigm, a willy-nilly eclecticism, or reductive versions of evidence-based practice, I have argued, we must formulate basic principles and values that guide our ways of working in the concrete particularity of the clinical situation.

As we have seen, the orienting perspectives of clinical pragmatism center on essential concerns widely believed to shape the course and outcomes of psychotherapy: our focus on the patient as an individual, subjective domains of experience, and notions of personal agency, freedom, and choice; the core conditions of the therapeutic relationship, collaboration, and the dynamics of interactive experience; open-ended dialogue and the co-creation of meaning and narratives that deepen understanding of self, life experience, and anticipated future; pluralist approaches to understanding, guided by scientific reasoning and humanistic values, that offer plausible ways of formulating what is the matter and what carries the potential to help; varied opportunities for experiential learning, fostering a sense of mastery and the development of capacities and skills, and ongoing assessment of progress and outcomes over the course of the therapeutic process.

The fundamental ethical value of clinical pragmatism lies in the practical outcomes of help and care, as Brendel (2006), Goldberg (2002), and Strenger (1997) emphasize in their accounts. We consider a range of paradigms and perspectives as we work to understand the patient, problems in living, and what carries the potential to help, taking account of differences in personality and temperament, the nature of subjective experience, capacities and skills, experiential learning and the irreducible features of the therapeutic process that defy classification.

Although advances in clinical neuroscience and psychopharmacology at the end of the 20th century had moved some scholars to predict that biomedical models of explanation and treatment would supplant the practice of psychotherapy, as noted in earlier discussions, ongoing research on neuroplasticity reaffirms the crucial role of established psychological and social practices in our efforts to bring about change, growth, and healing. The brain is far more plastic than modern neuroscientists had once assumed, and we increasingly appreciate the critical role of relational life and experiential learning in change and growth. Diverse forms of activity and learning carry the potential to change the brain and mind across the course of life.

We have explored the ways in which recent developments in interpersonal neurobiology deepen our appreciation of subjectivity, relationship, narrative, life experience, and different forms of therapeutic action in accord with the principles of clinical pragmatism. If we consider the neural substrates of the "talking cure," I observed in the Introduction, a fundamental task of psychotherapy is to generate experiential opportunities that strengthen the integration and regulation of neural structures and functions thought to underlie our sense of self, well-being, and adaptive functioning. In accord with continued research in the fields of neurogenetics, molecular biology, and brain imaging, the experiential changes we see over the course of psychotherapy would appear to be closely linked with changes in the structure and function of the brain.

Drawing on conceptual syntheses and empirical findings in interpersonal neurobiology, psychotherapy research, and clinical observation, we explored overlapping domains of experience that would appear to be fundamental in enhancing neuroplasticity, validating concepts of therapeutic action across the schools of thought. We focused on: 1) the core conditions of the therapeutic relationship, the dynamics of interactive experience, and the constancy of care in the holding environment; 2) the experience of emotion, challenge, and optimal stress; 3) the recurring engagement of sensation, emotion, imagery, cognition, and behavior in the interactive experience of the "working through" process, believed to facilitate the reorganization and growth of under-developed or under-regulated neural networks in accord with the dynamics of long-term potentiation; 4) the co-creation of narratives, synthesizing our experience of sensation, emotion, imagery, thought, and memory, strengthening coherence and unity in sense of self and identity; and 5) engagement of relationships, activities, practices, and places in everyday life.

Our reviews of the paradigms of psychotherapy deepen our appreciation of core processes believed to operate across all forms of treatment, as well as specific methods of intervention developed within particular schools of thought; as discussed, some researchers propose that different approaches engage different neuroanatomical structures instrumental in our experience of sensation, emotion, imagery, thought, and action. Converging lines of study in the science of mind emphasize the need to consider multiple theories, therapeutic languages, and technical procedures as we carry out "experiments in adapting to need," creating diverse forms of experiential learning in flexible, integrative ways of working.

While recent developments in the fields of neuroscience reaffirm the fundamental importance of theoretical pluralism and comparative approaches in therapeutic practice, as discussed, clinical training programs in psychiatry, psychology, counseling, and social work continue to marginalize theory, often limiting content to cognitive-behavioral perspectives. Many educators embrace reductive models of evidence-based treatment, emphasizing empirical research, technical procedures, and mastery of skills rather than comparative study of clinical theories that provide foundations for critical thinking, experiments in adapting to need, and individual approaches to practice.

The principles and values of clinical pragmatism challenge educators to expand the scope of clinical training. As we have seen, the foundational schools of thought set forth compelling accounts of the human situation, focusing our attention on overlapping realms of experience from different points of view, offering a variety of metaphors, languages, narratives, models, and methods that influence what we observe, say, and do in the clinical situation. Without a grounding in the foundational theories of the field, I have argued, we run the risk of reductive, mechanized approaches to treatment by protocol, unable to negotiate the complexities of the clinical situation, failing to understand the elements we are trying to integrate. As discussed, we may underestimate the potential benefits of different ways of working over the course of the therapeutic process, just as we may fail to appreciate the power of more focused, circumscribed approaches.

In accord with Dewey's emphasis on the critical role of collaboration in learning, understanding, and growth, I have emphasized the importance of ongoing dialogue across the fields of neuroscience, psychology, and the humanities. As we explore different ways of attending, understanding, and acting, we discover shared concerns and purposes, deepening our appreciation of the varieties of therapeutic experience. As James reminds us, the world is full of "partial purposes" and "partial stories"—"one" in some respects, "many" in others (1911, p. 134). As we carry out our work, he shows us, we can never make the big claim from a fixed point of reference. The fundamental question is not "Is it true?" but rather, how would our lives be better if we were to believe it?

References

Barlow, D. H., Allen, L. B. & Basden, S. L. (2007). Psychological treatments for panic disorders, phobias, and generalized anxiety disorder, in P. E. Nathan & J. M. Gorman (Eds.), *A guide to treatments that work*, 3rd edn (pp. 351–394). New York: Oxford University Press.

Borden, W. (2009). *Contemporary psychodynamic theory and practice*. New York: Oxford University Press.

Brendel, D. (2006). *Healing psychiatry: Bridging the science/humanism divide*. Cambridge, MA: MIT Press.

Cozolino, L. (2017). *The neuroscience of psychotherapy*, 3rd edn. New York: Norton.

Eigen, M. (1981/1993). The area of faith in Winnicott, Lacan and Bion, in A. Phillips (Ed.), *The electrified tightrope* (pp. 109–138). Northvale, NJ. Jason Aronson.

Goldberg, A. (2002). American pragmatism and American psychoanalysis. *Psychoanalytic Quarterly*, 71, 235–254.

James, W. (1911). The one and the many, in *Some problems of philosophy: A beginning of an introduction to philosophy* (pp. 113–146). New York: Longmans, Green.

Kantor, J. (1990). Community-based treatment of the psychotic client: The contributions of D. W. and Clare Winnicott. *Clinical Social Work Journal*, 18 (1), 23–41.

Ogden, T. (1986). *Matrix of the mind*. Northvale, NJ: Jason Aronson.

Sacks, O. (2019). *Everything in its place*. New York: Knopf.

Strenger, C. (1997). Hedgehogs, foxes, and critical pluralism. *Psychoanalysis and Contemporary Thought*, 20 (1), 111–145.

Van der Kolk, B. (2014). *The body keeps the score: Brain, mind, and body in the healing of trauma*. New York: Penguin.

Wallin, D. (2007). *Attachment in psychotherapy*. New York: Guilford.

Winnicott, D. W. (1947/1975). Hate in the countertransference, in D. W. Winnicott, *Through pediatrics to psycho-analysis* (pp. 194–203). New York: Basic.

Winnicott, D. W. (1960/1965). The theory of the parent-infant relationship, in D. W. Winnicott, *The maturational processes and the facilitating environment* (pp. 37–55). New York: International Universities Press.

Winnicott, D. W. (1962/1965). Ego integration in child development, in D. W. Winnicott, *The maturational processes and the facilitating environment* (pp. 56–63). New York: International Universities Press.

Winnicott, D. W. (1963/1965). The mentally ill in your caseload, in D. W. Winnicott, *The maturational processes and the facilitating environment* (pp. 217–229). Madison, CT: International Universities Press.

Winnicott, D. W. (1968/1987). Communication between infant and mother, and mother and infant, compared and contrasted, in C. Winnicott, R. Shepherd & M. Davis (Eds.), *D. W. Winnicott, babies and mothers* (pp. 89–103). Reading, MA: Addison Wesley.

Winnicott, D. W. (1971). *Playing and reality*. London: Tavistock.

Winnicott, D. W. (1988). *Human nature*. New York: Schocken Books.

Index

acceptance 62, 122, 123, 124, 136, 144
acceptance and commitment therapy
124–5; *see also* Hayes, Steven
accommodation 121–2, 141
active interventions 109, 122, 127, 159
activity and experiential learning 13, 14,
83–4; 109, 122, 129; see also clinical
pragmatism; pragmatism and American
philosophy
actualizing tendency, and Kurt Goldstein
153; and Carl Rogers 158
Addams, Jane 13, 93
Adler, Alfred 89, 101
adverse childhood events, and
attachment 45
agency, sense of, and behavioral paradigm
122, 124; and case study 176; and
clinical pragmatism 17, 18, 182;
and cognitive paradigm 136; and
humanistic paradigm 150, 156,
165; and psychodynamic paradigm
107–8, 111
Ainsworth, Mary 92
amygdala system: overview 41; and
implicit memory 46–7; and
neural integration 43, 47–8; and
orbitoprefrontal cortex and right
hemisphere 43, 54
analytical psychology, and neuroscience
80–2; and personality development
80–2; and self 82; and therapeutic
action 83–4
Anna O. 74–5; *see also* Pappenheim,
Bertha
arts and therapeutic action 61, 63, 111
assimilation, 121–2, 141
attachment: and Bowlby, John 92–3; and
development of the brain, overview
43–5; and dynamics of interactive

experience 43–4; empirical research
43–5, 92–3; and psychopathology and
adverse health outcomes 44–5; and
psychotherapy 44–5, 60–1; and
interactive regulation of self states
43–5; and right cerebral hemisphere
44–5; and Schore, Allan 43–5; and
trauma 44–5, 170–3
attending, ways of, and nature of experience
5; *see also* McGilchrist, Iain
attunement, and dynamics of attachment
43–5; and therapeutic action 19, 94,
97–8, 106–7, 157, 161; *see also*
humanistic paradigm; psychodynamic
paradigm; self psychology
Atwood, George 101; *see also* unconscious
processes
autonomic nervous system, and neural
development 39–40; and trauma, 40;
see also fight, flight or freeze response;
parasympathetic branch of nervous
system; sympathetic branch of
nervous system

Bandura, Albert 119
Barlow, David, and panic disorder
170; and process-based therapy
120; psychological treatments *vs.*
psychotherapy 128
Beck, Aaron 135, 137–9; see also
behavioral paradigm; cognitive
paradigm
Beebe, Beatrice 98
behavioral activation 127; and case
study 172
behavioral paradigm 116–131; and
case studies 170–78; and clinical
pragmatism 128, 129–30; and
cognitive paradigm, 116, 119, and

evolution of therapeutic practice 118–120; models 120–5; neuroscience and therapeutic action 128–9; origins 117–18; and psychodynamic paradigm 107; and therapeutic action 125–8

belief, and placebo effect 21–22

Berlin, Sharon 137, 140–1

bilateral integration 54–5; *see also* narrative; left cerebral hemisphere; right cerebral hemisphere

Binswanger, Ludwig 153

Blagys, Matthew 71–2

Bleuler, Eugen 79

bodily sensation and experiential domains of therapeutic action 159–60, 161, 162, 164; *see also* Gendlin, Eugene; Greenberg, Leslie; humanistic paradigm; interoceptive attention

body, somatic markers and subjectivity 40; and neural development 52; *see also* Damasio, Antonio

body, right brain to right brain intersubjectivity 44, 60–1

Bollas, Christopher, and unthought known 101

borderline personality disorder, and case study, 173–8; and neuroscience 45, 174–5, 180; and therapeutic action 173–8

Boss, Medard 153

bottom-up processes,42, 53–4, 56; and therapeutic action 56–7, 63, 110, 129, 164

Bowlby, John 44, 92–3; *see also* attachment theory

brain, anatomy and function, overview 36–43; and attachment 43–5; compared to mind 36; connectivity 39, 43, 52; connectome 39; defined 36; and laterality 41–2, 54–5; and memory 46–8; and narrative 41–2; and neural development 37–8; and neuroplasticity 37, 38, 57–60; *see also* left cerebral hemisphere; right cerebral hemisphere

brain stem, overview 39–40

Brendel, David, and clinical pragmatism xiii, 14, 16, 18, 182; on mind-body problem and non-reductive materialism 35–6

Breuer, Josef, and emotion 61; and trauma 74–5

Broca, Pierre Paul 54

Bruner, Jerome 135

Buddhism, and science of mind 134; and therapeutic action 120, 123, 134, 137

Cajal, Santiago Ramon y, and neural doctrine 37–8; and neuroplasticity 37, 39; and theory of dynamic polarization 37

case management, and D. W. Winnicott 175–6, 177

case studies: Jonathan 167–73; Marta 173–8; and principles and values of clinical pragmatism 178–84

Cassirer, Ernst 133

cerebral cortex, overview 41–3

Chalmers, David, and consciousness 34

Charcot, Jean-Martin 74–5, 79

Churchland, Patricia S., and reductive materialism 33–4

Churchland, Paul M. and reductive materialism 33–4

classical conditioning 118, 122

clinical pragmatism, and individuality 17–18; and neuroscience 63–4, 182–3; and pluralist orientation 19, 180–1; principles and values 16–22, 178–84; and reflection-in-action, experiential learning, and practical outcomes 22, 179, 181; and relationship and collaboration 18–19, 179; and subjectivity 17–18; and therapeutic outcomes 25, 182–3; and training 183

cognitive behavior therapy, empirical research and brain function 145

cognitive paradigm 133–149; case studies 171–8; and clinical pragmatism 147; constructivist perspective 136–7, 142–4; and emotion 143–4; and evolution of therapeutic practice 133–7; integrative perspective 140–1; models 137–41; neuroscience and therapeutic action 144–6; origins 133–4; rationalist perspective 134–5, 141–2; and therapeutic action 141–4

cognitive revolution 116, 119, 134, 135

Coles, Robert xii; and humanities 20; and narrative 20, 107

connectome 39, 55

consciousness, and experience 38; and mind-body relationship 33–6; *see also* Dewey, John; James, William

constructivist models of cognitive therapy 136–7, 139–40, 142–3

context, and behavioral paradigm 119, 121, 126; and John Dewey 14